TELL ME ABOUT IT

MEMOIR OF A PSYCHOTHERAPIST

PINNY BRAKELEY BUGAEFF
MSW, LCSW

Copyright © Pinny Brakeley Bugaeff, MSW, LCSW, 2018

Produced by Ant Press: www.antpress.org

First Edition

The author asserts the moral right under the Copyright, Designs and Patents Act 1988 to be identified as the author of this work.

All rights reserved. No part of this publication may be reproduced, stored in a retrieval system, or transmitted, in any form or by any means without the prior written consent of the author, nor be otherwise circulated in any form of binding or cover other than that in which it is published and without a similar condition being imposed on the subsequent purchaser.

In order to protect the sacred bond of confidentiality that is forged when a client chooses to open themselves to the therapeutic process, names, gender, occupations, locations, dates, events, and all other potential identifying details have been changed, but, at the heart of each story, is truth.

DEDICATION

For Alex, the love of my life, who believed in me long before I came to believe in myself and who encouraged me, over and over, to tell my story. You are still the best thing that ever happened to me.

For my son, Gregor, Sculptor Extraordinaire, you gave me a lifelong gift—the courage to follow you on your journey along the Artist's Way.

For my daughter, Mandy, Teacher of the Year—I see who I want to be in the ways you love and live your life.

PREFACE

Let's face it. What kind of kid wants to be a psychotherapist when they grow up? Who dreams of spending their days sitting in a beige room, listening to an unending litany of pain? Not me. I was going to be a cowboy. Blaze, my Palomino stallion, and I were going to spend our days chasing varmints and rounding up strays. Come sundown, we'd pitch camp in a cottonwood grove and rustle up some grub. Then, lulled by the faraway sound of the Sons of the Pioneers crooning, "Happy Trails to You," we'd fall asleep under the stars.

However, before I could saddle up, I hit the perfect pre-therapist–in-training trifecta. First, my father—smart, funny, and kind—was alcoholic. Second, my beautiful mother, although wildly creative, suffered from a mood disorder. And third, at the age of eight, I was molested by a stranger.

So, like many of the other therapists I know, I started my field training early on, in the bosom of my family, facing the issues one is most likely to encounter in the world of the disordered and distressed: addiction, mental illness, and sexual abuse.

Truthfully, many of us entered the field to try and understand what had happened to us and how we could heal ourselves. In retrospect, my early life experiences laid a foundation for me to give meaning to the pain and despair of my childhood and gave me a lifelong motivation to try and help others find their way out of the darkness. As much as I may have helped my clients on their journey to healing, I received far more than I gave.

CONTENTS

1. Playing the Cat	1
2. What's Past is Prologue	7
3. Whirly Gig	13
4. California Dreamin'	25
5. Brokenhearted	31
6. The Mad Millionaire, M.D.	45
7. Crash and Burn	51
8. I Spy	55
9. Love Story	63
10. Rip-off	81
11. God Help Us	87
12. Kenny the Farting Angel	99
13. Gotta Buy a Rat	111
14. Lady Godiva	117
15. Tiger, Tiger Burning Bright	127
16. We're Baaaaack	133
17. Tell Me a Story	135
18. Kid in a Cage	145
19. Milo the Sumo	151
Afterword	157
Contact the Author	159
Acknowledgments	161

1
PLAYING THE CAT

State Hospital—Forensic Hold Unit

The information on the hospital intake report was scanty. Lillian Stubbs, age 72, had, the previous night, gotten out of bed, grabbed a souvenir Red Sox bat off the mantle, and bashed in the brains of her sleeping husband, Ralph. After she called the police, she was booked and transported to the forensic ward of the state hospital.

Mrs. Stubbs was being held on suicide watch in the observation room. I made my way down the bile green hallway and through the double set of locked doors that led to the Forensic Hold Unit. Expecting to see a wild-eyed woman sunk into despair, I peeked through the small observation window of her room. Lillian, puffy gray hair piled in a bun, wearing wire-rimmed spectacles, was sitting quietly on the edge of the iron bed, hands folded in her lap. She was the spitting image of Granny from the Tweety Bird and Sylvester cartoons.

When I'd read the police report, I'd have been willing to bet that the impetus for her bloody act of homicide must have been a severe psychiatric disorder. But, given her demeanor, it took a second to readjust my assumptions.

Stan, the unit orderly, unlocked Lillian's door.

"Mrs. Stubbs," I said.

"Yes," she answered in a little-girl voice which was at odds in a woman of her age. It's been my experience that, sometimes, when a female client speaks in a childish or baby-like voice, she may have a history of sexual abuse. I mentally filed that thought for a later interview. Lots of women have high-pitched voices, and other types of early trauma can trigger behaviors that are inexplicable—like a seemingly happily married grandma bashing in her husband's skull with a baseball bat.

I spent the first half hour getting Lillian's history and building rapport. Then asked her, "Lillian, can you tell me why you killed Ralph?"

"He wouldn't stop playing the cat."

She said it just like that, as if she were talking about slapping a pesky mosquito.

"What? How do you mean, 'playing with the cat?'" Given her mild manner, it was hard for me to understand why she'd kill her husband for playing with the cat.

"Not playing *with* the cat," she said. "Playing the cat. Every time he got liquored up, he'd grab my cat, jam her head under his elbow, and squeeze till she'd start yowling, then he'd march around the house, pretending to play her like a bagpipe. I begged him to stop but...enough is enough."

Enough is enough. Probably the clearest, most succinct motivation for behavior I'd ever heard. Lillian spent four months in the hospital, then, due to her age and lack of any other criminal or aggressive behavior, it was decided at her court hearing that there was little likelihood of Lillian bashing anyone else. (Well, unless some poor fool decided to play the cat like a bagpipe.) Her attorney made a plea deal and she was sentenced to confinement at the hospital for six months.

Over the next few months, I got to know Lillian pretty well. During a later session, I asked her if there had ever been abuse when she was growing up.

"Abuse?" she answered in her little-girl voice. "Like what kind of abuse?"

"Well, there's physical abuse, like pinching or slapping or spanking. There's mental abuse, calling you bad names or screaming at you or making you feel ashamed of yourself. There's sexual abuse, like someone who touches you or kisses you in a way that makes you feel uncomfortable or…" Before I finished the question, Lillian's affect changed. A deep red flush crawled up her neck and flooded her face with crimson. She stared at the floor as she began to talk.

"Well, my older cousin, Charles," she hesitated, then in her little-girl voice said, "made me play…ummm…games." She glanced up at me over the top of her spectacles, checking to see how I was taking this information. I nodded encouragement for her to continue.

"Well…" She was blushing furiously. "You know…made me… touch him and…" I waited for her to say more, but she stared at the floor, perhaps replaying the unspeakable.

"How old were you?"

"Maybe four or five," she answered in her whispery, little-girl voice.

"How old was your cousin?"

"I think he was twelve or so."

"Did anybody ever find out? Did you tell anyone?"

Lillian looked up at me as if I were a moron. (Given my decision about my own similar experience, I understood.)

"*No.*" The little-girl voice disappeared. She lifted her head and looked me in the eye. "He said if I told, he'd kill my dog."

My inner dialogue was starting to crank up. I admit to a moment of fantasizing mental murder of Charles. These days, it's PC to never say anything judgmental about anyone. For the politically correct, the worst that can be said about a child molester who commits emotional blackmail on a four-year-old by threatening to kill her pet is—He Made Poor Choices. Not that he was evil or perverse, just that he made poor choices.

A poor choice is eating all your Halloween candy at one sitting and getting a tummy ache. A poor choice is deciding to wash and wax the car even though the chance of rain is 80 percent. There are some things that are so hardwired, no amount of counseling, psychotherapy, or medication will help. Evil is one of those things. Pedophilia is another.

People scoff at the notion of evil. (Those of the Poor Choices School.) They seem to believe that, if someone just gets enough of the right kind of love, acceptance, and counseling, the person will transform. I've worked in environments where evil is the coin of the realm. I won't say that soul-deep transformation never happens, but, when it does, it borders on the miraculous. The most famous case that comes to mind is Saint Paul, former torturer of Christians, who was transformed on the road to Damascus.

Lillian looked so embarrassed, I almost decided to shift the conversation, but, truthfully, it was I who was not comfortable. Given my own history, sexual abuse of children is one of those areas where my compassion for the perp wanes. I understand that many abusers were victims themselves, and luckily there are a lot of other therapists who do have the stomach for working with molesters. In any case, hearing about what had happened to Lillian and seeing her pain still palpable, even years later, triggered my experience with the guy on the beach who'd molested me. I'd spent a lot of hours in therapy, working toward integrating that experience, and I recognized I needed to dial everything back so Lillian didn't get caught up in my emotional undertow. This was Lillian's journey, not mine.

"Lillian, I'm so sorry you had to go through that. Did anyone ever find out what Charles did to you?"

"No." The little-girl voice faded, replaced by the voice of a grown woman.

"Do you ever see him at family gatherings?"

"No. Charles is dead."

I was at a crossroad. I could close this up or proceed and let her tell me her story. No contest.

"When did he die?"

"August fourth, 1916."

I was surprised she remembered the exact date. I was getting a funny twinge in my gut. "What happened to him?"

"We were there throwing rocks, and he fell off the quarry cliff," she said in a little-girl voice.

I hesitated. It wasn't just her answer; it was her affect and presentation. At that moment, I had a mental image of Charles standing at the edge of the quarry. One minute, he's bending over, picking up a rock, and, the next minute, he's flying through the air, headed for the massive blocks of stone at the bottom.

Ka-ching! Could it be? Was the lovely Lillian—Tweety's grandma—possibly on her way to being a serial killer? The common criteria to qualify as a serial killer is three people killed at different times in different places. She was two for two. Of course, I had no evidence she did anything like shove her cousin off the cliff. Everything was conjecture on my part. But, when I get that feeling in my gut, a lot of times I'm right. I erased my own little mentally murderous DVD and refocused on Lillian, who was sitting across from me, hands in her lap, no trace of guilt or shame, smiling serenely. She was 72 years old. The Charles incident had happened more than 60 years prior.

If Lillian *did* kill her cousin, I didn't have any proof. She was a model patient. Her sentence was almost up, and now she'd answered the one question—about Ralph, her husband, and the same answer as to why she may have shoved Charles off the cliff.

Enough is enough. Best explanation I'd heard in a long time.

The rest of the story

Here's the lifelong lesson I learned from Lillian: Looks can be deceiving.

2
WHAT'S PAST IS PROLOGUE

Looking back, I see that everything that happened to me before I became a psychotherapist was preparation for all that was to follow. I was blessed to live through events which, although they seemed traumatic at the time, gave me the experience of having walked in the shoes of many of my clients. And speaking of shoes…

I was born in 1942, with feet so radically turned inward the doctor was afraid I'd never walk normally. When I was about nine months old, he advised my mother to put me into special baby shoes—brown leather high-tops that were connected by a wide, metal spacer bar. He said the device would straighten my feet and knees and I'd learn to walk. Well, despite the shoes, or because of them, I did learn to walk. However, I'm still so pigeon-toed that strangers in the park scatter bird seed on the sidewalk when I walk by.

The first house I remember living in was a three-story Victorian in Plainfield, N.J. My bedroom had a fireplace, and my dad would come in early in the morning to light a fire and hang my clothes in front of it so they were warm when I got dressed. My great-grandmother, Gan, stayed in a tiny bedroom next to mine. Most mornings, she'd come in to get me dressed, then we'd wend our way down the long, winding staircase where my mother, a Georgia Peach from Savannah, would present us with a sumptuous breakfast: grits with ham or maybe corncakes or sausage. After breakfast, Gan would wash the dishes, and my dad, a chemist, would leave for work. My brother, Peter, three years older than I, who was a brain and taught himself to read before he went to kindergarten, would leave for a mythic place called school, and I'd be left to my own devices. Although I was only four, and my mother told me to stay in the yard, I liked exploring the neighborhood.

So, frequently, when my mother looked outside to check on me, I'd be gone. Naturally, she'd come unhinged until she found me up a tree or down the street next to the lake, watching the ducks. Her solution to that problem today would have earned her a visit from a Child Protection Agency, but then it must have seemed like a practical solution to tie a rope around my waist and attach the other end to the overhead clothesline with a snap clip; that way, I could still run around the yard but not run away and get lost.

At first, it was kind of fun. I galloped up and down the yard, pretending I was a wild pony, but that got old. So I sat down under the lilac tree one day and went to work untying the knot around my waist. It didn't take long before the rope fell off. I snuck between the hedge and the side of the house and stopped at the edge of the front porch. The coast was clear. I ran down the street to the corner, made sure to look both ways, and waited for the light to go green. Next thing I knew, a policeman came running toward me.

"Hey! You!" he yelled.

I stopped for a second and looked around. I was pretty sure he wasn't yelling at me. I'd looked both ways before crossing. I'd waited for a green light. So...

"Hey...little girl. Stop."

Oh boy. A policeman was calling me. I knew I was in big trouble—gonna-get-a-spanking trouble. I started to cry.

"Aw." He bent down on one knee. "Don't cry. Yer mother's looking for you."

Just then, my mother appeared. My Georgia Peach, charming, petite, blond mother who laid it on thick.

"Oh, officer, thank God. Ah was just about to lose mah mind."

I wasn't fooled. As soon as the cop was gone, she was going to drag me home and snatch me baldheaded. And she did just that. Wasn't the first time and for sure wouldn't be the last.

Four years later, when I was eight, my baby sister, Polly, was born, and we moved to a resort town at the Jersey shore. At the end of August, the tourists left, and the other townie kids and I were free to roam. We'd leave the house in the morning, run home for lunch, then run back outside to play until sunset.

Except, one summer morning, before anyone else was awake, I snuck out of the house. It was a block from the beach, and I wanted to get there early, before the other kids arrived, so I could finish digging out the sand dune cave we'd started the day before. I ran down to the end of the block and arrived at the beach just in time to see the sunrise flood the sky with light. I stood for a minute, watching the sandpipers playing tag with the waves. Then I grabbed the little trenching shovel out of the cave and started digging.

"Pretty morning, ain't it?"

Startled, I whirled around. A young guy, maybe seventeen or eighteen, was standing at the bottom of the dune. I got a sinking feeling in the pit of my stomach.

He pointed to the sky. "That sky is almost as pretty as you."

I wanted to run, but something told me not to.

"I'll give you a dollar for kiss," he said.

I had no way to process what he was saying, except some kind of atavistic fear told me I was in deep trouble. He took a few steps toward me. I froze when he squatted down on his knees and pushed me into the half-dug cave.

"Close your eyes," he snarled, "and keep 'em closed."

He smelled like sweat and garlic. Time stood still. I went away someplace in my mind until I felt something warm splatter my face. My eyes flew open. I saw...

"Shut your eyes," he growled. I squeezed them tightly shut. I heard him zip his zipper.

I stayed in the cave for a long time then bolted out and ran down to the edge of the ocean. I threw myself face down in the shallow surf and frantically scrubbed off the slime with sand and sea water. Dripping wet, I stood and struggled back up to the beach.

Right then, I knew I was never going to tell anybody about the disgusting thing I'd allowed to be done to me. First of all, I'd get a spanking for sneaking out of the house and, second of all, I didn't have the language to describe exactly what had occurred. Back then, there was no such thing as "Stranger Danger" or "Bad Touch, Good Touch." I ran back home and made up a story to tell my mother why I was soaking wet. And never went to the beach alone again.

My penchant for "exploring" often led me down dark pathways, and yet I've always emerged alive. As I now read the sentence "finish digging out the sand dune cave," my blood runs cold. I read the words "pushed me into the half-dug cave," and feel the same chill. I've lived in big cities and worked with a variety of unpredictable and sometimes dangerous people and, until a few months before I retired, I was never harmed or injured. I call it the grace of God and am certain I have a full-time Guardian Angel.

SADLY, MY DAD'S DRINKING, COUPLED WITH MY MOTHER'S VOLATILE temperament, eventually led to divorce. My brother was sent to boarding school, and my mother moved with my sister and me into an apartment in Princeton, New Jersey.

I finished high school, determined to go as far away from Jersey as I could get. I applied to Whittier College in California and was accepted with a scholarship. I spent two years there, hanging out in the drama department and dating surfer dudes. But, deep down, I knew that, if I was ever going to get an education, I needed to stop playing around and buckle down.

I returned to New Jersey and took off the fall semester; time to refocus on my goals and to save up some money for school. I was lucky to find a job right away in a laundry, working the counter from 7:00 a.m. to 3:00 p.m., taking in the dirty laundry and putting away the clean laundry bundles that were stored in massive racks behind the counter. Since I got off work at three, I figured I could also handle a night-time job and earn twice as much money, twice as fast. I found a job working 4:00 p.m. to 11:00 p.m. in a soda shop. The seeds of workaholism were beginning to sprout.

That summer, through an old family friend, I got a job as a youth worker in New York City. The friend, a social worker with a New York agency, told me I'd be working with needy girls in the City. The details of the job were sketchy. I imagined working in what used to be called a settlement house, where I'd teach crafts and supervise jump rope contests for underprivileged kids. Imagine my surprise when I discovered I was to begin my journey working in the New York City Juvenile Hall.

3
WHIRLY GIG

Summer of '62. New York City

Dripping with sweat from the long, hot walk from the subway, I arrived for my first day of work at Spofford Hall, New York City's main detention center for delinquent boys. I had a hard time convincing the guard at the gate that I was the new worker, maybe because I was a five-foot-three, freckle-faced kid, wearing a yellow cotton dress, white sandals, and a daisy-print headband. Barely twenty, I looked about twelve.

The shift supervisor came out to see what the fuss was about. She unlocked the gate, ushered me into the main receiving area, handed me a ring of keys, and told me I'd be working at Manida Street, the girls' detention unit, located around the corner from Spofford.

On that first day, I was assigned to the "blockhouse," literally a one-story, flat-roofed building made of concrete block. Separated from the girls' main building and enclosed by a twelve-foot, chain-link fence, it stood by itself in the middle of a black-topped exercise yard. The supervisor led me across the yard and buzzed for the guard. A huge, African-American guy, his head shaved bald, appeared. He wore a black T-shirt, and his arm muscles were the size of bocce balls. He unlocked the barred door, looked at the director, then pointed at me.

"That's the new worker?" His tone implied this was some kind of joke.

The supervisor said, "Miss Brakeley, this is Mr. Glad. I'm sure he'll be glad to show you around." Mr. Glad gave a humorless snort at her lame pun. That introduction was the extent of the training I received.

Mr. Glad, who I later learned was a former semi-pro football player, led me into the day room—cinderblock walls painted flat gray and one window screened with heavy metal mesh. The only décor—a hand-drawn picture of a Valentine heart pierced with a knife—was taped to the wall. Six or seven girls of varying sizes, colors, and ages were scattered around the barren room. There was a small, square table bolted to the floor and two or three chairs, likewise bolted to the floor. At the far end of the room, the bathroom door stood halfway open.

Two of the girls were sitting at the table, one was braiding another girl's hair, and three others were sitting on the floor, playing jacks. They all stopped what they were doing and stared when I entered the room.

Back then, it was pretty much assumed that, if you got sent to juvie, you'd done something illegal. In fact, many of the girls there had only committed status offenses, which, in legal terms, means a noncriminal act that's considered a law violation only because the youth is a minor. Typical status offenses included truancy, running away from home, violating curfew, underage drinking, and behaviors beyond the control of a parent. Those girls lived in the main housing unit. However, as I soon found out, the girls in the blockhouse were not status offense kids. Most of them had committed a variety of criminal offenses like assault with a deadly weapon or homicide.

"Girls," Mr. Glad rumbled, "this is Miss Brakeley. You all don't give her any trouble, and she'll treat you right."

One of the girls cracked, "Yeah, she better." Everybody

laughed. Mr. Glad pulled me aside and, pointing at each girl, told me her street name: Phyllis, about five foot nine inches, maybe 180 pounds, wore a black do-rag bandanna; Poco, about four foot two inches, café au lait skin, jade green eyes; Sister wore an afro comb in her wild, black hair; Gypsy, about five foot eleven inches, easily 200 pounds; Poco, Lil'bit, and Eve all looked like they were no more than twelve or thirteen.

Back in the day, I had a good memory for faces, and I made a special effort to remember each girl's name. When Mr. Glad was done, I just stood there, because I had no idea what I was supposed to do. He signaled me to follow him into the tiny, glassed-in office located beside the entry door. He lowered his voice. "Listen, you gotta be careful not to let one of them get you alone in the bathroom. They have to ask permission to go, and you gotta unlock the door."

I must have looked confused, because the bathroom door was hanging halfway open.

"But it's unlocked."

"Yeah, but...the last lady worked here—Miss Fazey—they shoved her head in the toilet and gave her a whirly."

"A whirly?"

He looked at me like I was stupid. "A whirly...they hold your head underwater in the toilet and flush."

"So, we leave it unlocked?"

He rolled his eyes. "Yeah, unless the inspectors are here."

I wanted to be cool. I wanted to look like this whole thing was no big deal. I'm pretty sure I failed. Mr. Glad left the enclosure and announced "rec time." He unlocked the door to the black-topped yard, and the girls straggled out. A few went to shoot baskets. Two of the girls wandered over to me.

"Hey, Gypsy...Poco..." I greeted them. Poco stopped short.

"How you know me?"

I am blessed, or, some might say, cursed, with a fast mouth. I said the first thing that came to mind.

"Poco, you're unforgettable."

She cracked up.

Gypsy said, "You are *so* right." Our laughter brought over two more girls. I greeted them by name. "Phyllis, Sister, nice of you two to join us."

In a belligerent voice, Phyllis asked Poco and Gypsy, "What's so funny?"

Gypsy answered, "The lady said Poco was unforgettable."

Phyllis snickered. "She got that right." She was a tall, African-American girl, about fourteen. She'd been sent from the main building to the blockhouse, because she'd shoved one of the youth workers in the main building down three flights of stairs. Phyllis's original charge was related to stabbing her father to death. (When I learned what he'd done to her, I have to admit I didn't blame her.) The murder charge definitely wasn't a status offense.

It took a second to register that Poco referred to me as "the lady."

"Uh...my last name is kind of tricky. How 'bout you call me Miss B?"

Gypsy asked, "Where you from?"

I recognized I was getting into sticky territory by answering personal questions, but, since I had no idea what I was doing, I kept it brief. "Jersey. How about you all?"

Phyllis chimed in. "I got an aunt in Jersey."

When the conversation devolved into whose auntie, godmother, or sister lived where, I breathed a sigh of relief.

Mr. Glad blew a whistle, and we went back to the blockhouse where we found a pile of brown-paper lunch bags stacked on the table. Everybody grabbed one. Four girls sat at the table and the others on the floor. Mr. Glad motioned me over.

"The girls get bag lunches, but we send out for lunch. What do you want? Pizza?"

Oh, boy. I was famished, but I wasn't about to sit down in front of the girls, who were eating thin bologna sandwiches on white bread, while I scarfed up something really tasty.

"Um, I ate late; I'm not really hungry…"

"Okay, suit yourself," he said. The unit doorbell rang. Mr. Glad went over and had a brief conversation with the guy at the door. Later, I spotted Mr. Glad in the office, slurping up a slice of pizza.

My shift ended at 4:00 p.m. I trudged down Longwood Avenue to catch the subway back to my apartment in Greenwich Village. I was shell-shocked. I'd imagined my job would involve playing jump rope and weaving lanyards, but, instead, I'd landed inside a jail for kids. Granted, it was fascinating, but I felt woefully underequipped to deal with what my old family friend had euphemistically described as "needy girls."

I slogged down the stairs to the subway platform and let myself be carried by the tide of wilted workers onto the waiting train. There were no seats, so I stood, hanging onto a pole, all the way to my stop on Christopher Street. I could hardly wait to get back to the apartment I'd sublet for the summer on West 11th Street.

At that time, Greenwich Village was really more like a small town rather than a neighborhood in New York City. A canopy of trees shaded cobblestone streets. Small mom-and-pop stores displayed their wares on sidewalk stalls. On the walk back to my apartment, I passed the outdoor flower stand. The fragrance from the blossoms mingled with the spicy smell of pizza and undernotes of bus fumes was, to me, the perfume of the city.

My apartment was a one-room, basement studio, about eighteen feet long by about eight feet wide. It had no real kitchen, except for a hotplate and a tiny old fridge, and the bathroom lacked a shower or a tub. No problem. After I moved in, I bought an inflatable, Mickey Mouse, kiddie wading pool and a garden hose. Every night before bed, I'd blow up the kiddie pool and set it on the bathroom floor. Then I'd crawl out my window and attach the hose to the faucet just outside the window. I'd feed the hose into my room, turn on the spigot, fill the tub, loll around in the nice cool water, and wash up.

That night, after I fed the hose back out the window, used a coffee can to bail the water from the pool into the sink, and deflated the pool, I fell into bed and lay awake. What I had gotten myself into? Somehow, while I slept, self-doubt dissolved. I woke up filled with resolve, determined to rise to the challenge of caring for what I now thought of as my girls.

THE NEXT MORNING, I ARRIVED AT THE FACILITY, AND MR. BAGLEY, the director, called me into his office. "Since you're a temporary worker, you're designated as a Special Police Lieutenant." Well, that didn't make any sense at all. My job title was Youth Worker. When I asked him about it, he shrugged and said, "That's the way the City wants it."

I never did figure out how I came to achieve that status, but one of my prized possessions that summer was the small, black leather flip case he gave me. It held a shiny gold police badge with blue enamel embossing that said Special Police Lieutenant. I became quite adept at flipping it open to show to the subway guards who would then open a special gate so that I could take whichever girl I was escorting onto the subway.

As it turned out, the major part of my job was to escort the girls to their court hearings and medical appointments. There are five boroughs in New York City, and, most mornings, I would go to the office and get my assignment as to which girl I was to escort, either to court or to a medical or psychiatric appointment.

Usually, a driver in a state car came to pick us up, and we'd arrive with little fuss, but, sometimes, all the drivers were busy, so, if the hearing or appointment was in the Bronx or Manhattan, I'd handcuff the girl to me, and we'd walk to the subway. In retrospect, I must have been quite a sight, marching down 125th Street, handcuffed to a girl usually much taller and heftier than me, but New Yorkers tend to be jaded, and it takes more than the sight of two young women walking handcuffed down the avenue for them to really take notice. Once we arrived at the subway turnstiles, I'd flash my snazzy badge to the cop on duty, he'd swing open an access gate, and then I'd wait with my charge on the platform for the proper train to arrive.

I always wondered why nobody tried to run away. They knew I had the handcuff key; it wouldn't have been hard to knock me down, take the key, and take off. Only once did I get a hint that the idea of escape might be percolating. It was the middle of July, so hot the tar on the street was melting. Phyllis, the girl the size of a linebacker, and I were heading toward the subway station, on our way to Manhattan Court for a hearing on her murder charge.

"Miss B," she said with a sly smile, "what'd you do if I ran?"

I'd thought about that a lot and still didn't have a clue what I'd do except hope I wouldn't be dragged down the street like a Chihuahua on a leash. I said the first thing that came to mind.

"Phyllis, if you feel you have to run, you gotta give me a chance to undo the cuffs, 'cause it's just too hot to chase after you." There was a long pause. Then she laughed.

"Sheeet...ya got that right."

We trudged down the stairs to the subway gates. I flashed my badge to the cop on duty. He glanced down at the handcuffs that bound me to Phyllis. With disbelief in his eyes he said, "Geez, you sure is young to be a flatfoot." We pushed through the revolving gate and waited for the subway to arrive.

On another occasion, I had to take Phyllis to a psychiatric evaluation at Bellevue Hospital. Her trial for stabbing her father was coming up, and the public defender wanted a psychiatric evaluation for her. I wondered if the public defender was going to have Phyllis claim temporary insanity as a motive for the stabbing.

I'd gotten to know Phyllis a little since we spent so much time traveling together, and, in my book, she wasn't any sort of crazy. (I'm aware that crazy is no longer a politically correct term, but it was considered appropriate back then.) Over time, she'd told me that, not only had her father sexually abused her, but he was also abusing her nine-year-old sister, Maria, now in foster care. The stabbing happened when the father tried to force Phyllis to have oral sex with a guy he owed money to.

Bellevue Hospital, in the early '60s, renowned for its massive psychiatric unit, was almost literally Bedlam. Although it was the dawn of new psychotropic medications for the chronically mentally ill, those meds weren't usually available, and, on top of that, state mental hospitals were closing down, forcing many of these people to live on the streets.

Just trying to get into the clinic, we had to edge our way around three white-coated orderlies who were trying to wrestle a bag lady through the door while she was spitting and screaming obscenities.

Once inside the lobby, we entered a long, marble hall lined with wooden-backed benches filled with street people. Many sat mumbling curses. Homeless addicts wandered aimlessly, listlessly scratching themselves. Hookers in miniskirts sashayed around, trolling for customers or maybe just too wired to sit still.

Huge ceiling fans did nothing to cool, only served to spread the miasma of the unwashed evenly through the waiting room. Scattered among the hopeless and homeless was a smattering of well-dressed men and women who may or may not have been some of the "walking wounded," or maybe they were relatives. In any case, we made our way to the admission desk, checked in, then waited for Phyllis's name to be called.

Finally, it was her turn, and an orderly led us down another long hall to the office of Dr. Targon. We stopped at the door. The orderly knocked, and a voice from inside said, "Come."

"Got another one for ya, Doc," the orderly said.

Dr. Targon sat behind a battered desk piled with paper, books, charts, a grease-stained brown bag, and other detritus. Middle-aged, a little paunchy, he stood up and gestured for us to come in. He stuck out his hand to shake hands with Phyllis, but, since she was cuffed, both our hands came up together. He raised his eyebrows in surprise.

"What's this?" he asked and pointed to the cuffs.

I spoke up. "Hi, I'm a youth worker at Manida Street, and this is Phyllis. She's here for her psych eval, but we had to come by subway so…they make us cuff up."

"Hmmm." He frowned. "Can you take off the cuffs?"

"Not really. I know this is supposed to be a confidential interview…but…"

To my surprise, Phyllis spoke up. "Miss B can stay. I ain't got nothing to say she hasn't heard before."

The doctor nodded. "Okay, as long as it's okay with you."

He began the interview. "Phyllis," he said, "the court wants to know if I think you're crazy, which is why we're meeting today. But, first of all, do you have any questions for me?"

Phyllis looked down when she spoke. "Doc, maybe I am crazy, but you know what my poppi did, right?"

"Tell me."

Phyllis stared at him for a second. "You didn't read the papers and stuff?"

"I did read the papers, but what the papers say isn't always the whole story; that's why I want you to tell me your side."

Phyllis sounded skeptical. "Did the lawyer tell you what happened?"

Phyllis's public defender, a young woman fresh out of law school, seemed to be invested in helping her.

"She did. She was the one who asked for this evaluation."

"Does she think I'm crazy?"

"She doesn't think so. Do you think you're crazy?"

Phyllis spaced out for a moment and then said, "I just didn't want to do it anymore." She dropped her chin to her chest. Huge tears spattered down onto the gray linoleum floor and left tiny, wet puddles. She sat sobbing silently. I knew from experience how one learns to cry without making a sound. It takes a lot of practice.

Dr. Targon sat patiently, waiting for the storm to pass. He passed her a handful of tissues. She took them without looking at him. As she reached for them, she dragged our cuffed hands up, blew her nose, and wiped her face.

"What's 'it'?" he asked.

Phyllis rolled her eyes. "I didn't want him messin' with me anymore."

"Messin' how?"

Phyllis was getting an edge to her voice. "How do you think? What don't you understand about messin' with me?"

"Phyllis, I'm pretty sure I get your meaning, but I need for you to say it out loud so the court knows exactly why you did what you did."

Phyllis leaned forward, and spit flew from her mouth. "He was f--king me." She screamed at the doctor. "And he was startin' on Maria, and then he was gonna make me give Pedro a BJ. Now you get it?"

The doctor looked remarkably calm. "I get you loud and clear. I am so sorry he did that to you. Before you told me that, you looked so sad. What were the tears for?"

"I killed my father. I couldn't make him stop..." She began to cry again. "You know...I hated it when he started on Maria. Oh no...no more...but it was the BJ for Pedro that did it."

"The BJ for Pedro?"

"BJ—ya know what a BJ is?" The rage was boiling.

"I do. He wanted you to have oral sex with his friend? How old was Pedro?"

"How the hell I know? He was old."

Phyllis didn't actually worry about what was going to happen to her. One day on the way to her final hearing she said, "Least I got Maria outta there."

The rest of the story

Despite her attorney's pleas and Dr. Targon's evaluation, Phyllis was sent to Hudson Training School. Located in upper New York State, it was called a training school and was theoretically based on principles of instilling morals and values, but it was more like a prison farm for kids.

I wasn't at work on the evening they took Phyllis up to Hudson, but, the next morning, when I arrived, the girls came over and talked about seeing their friend taken away to serve four years for killing her father.

"Miss B, how come they send Phyllis to Hudson, but they didn't do nuthin' when her poppi was messin' with her an' her sister?"

I was sick at heart. I had no answer for her. I had the same question.

"Poco, I don't know. It's not fair. What do you think they should have done?"

"Sheeet...I think they shoulda cut his dick off." The girls all laughed. There seemed to be universal agreement that her suggestion was the right punishment for Poppi.

I still think about Phyllis. I wonder what happened to her and the thousands of other girls like her. I often wished I could tell her that my outrage about her story helped fuel the fire inside me to try to right some of the wrongs perpetrated against children.

Spofford Hall and Manida Street were closed long ago. And, although the knowledge base about child development and the treatment of at-risk youth has evolved, sadly, there is still a very long way to go.

4

CALIFORNIA DREAMIN'

At the end of the summer, my job in New York City ended, and I transferred to Drew, a small college in Madison, New Jersey. On the first day of the semester, I was sitting in the cafeteria with my roommate, Jean, a Courtney Cox type, except Jean wore horn-rimmed glasses and needed braces. I surveyed the motley assortment of young men and was happy to see that most of them were pale and scrawny and looked as dull as sheep—no chance here of male distractions.

I was on a mission—get my degree in social work and return as quickly as possible to the field. I took a sip of coffee and began studying for my upcoming sociology quiz.

I finished the chapter, closed the book, glanced across the room, and there, standing in the doorway, was the handsomest guy I'd ever seen. Tall, chiseled features, dark eyes—think a young Clint Eastwood. I was struck so hard, I saw stars and planets and little birdies. I felt like the cartoon version of Goofy falling in love.

"Who's that?" I asked.

"Oh yeah," Jean said, "don't get your hopes up. His name is Alex. He doesn't date any girls here."

I didn't say anything, but the thought balloon over my head read: *We'll see about that.*

Much later, Alex told me this: "I was sitting in the lounge with Peter, my roommate. We were waiting for lunch when you walked by on your way to the cafeteria. You were beautiful: long, blond hair, great build, you were wearing a suede dress and huarache sandals—my surfer-girl fantasy come to life. I asked Peter, 'Who's that?' 'That's the new girl from California,' he told me, 'but Jean says she's here to study and doesn't have any interest in going out with guys here.'"

The next day, I sat by myself at a little table in the cafeteria once again, studying. A shadow fell across the page. I looked up. Alex was smiling as he sat down across from me.

"Hi," he said, "I'm Alex." He glanced at my text book, which happened to be economics.

"So," he asked, "what d'you think about the European Common Market?"

Best come-on line ever. We talked for two hours.

"There's a party on Friday. D'you want to go?" he asked.

I barely registered what he said, because the little stars and planets and birdies circling my head were now accompanied by strains of violins playing "Moon River."

On Friday night, he picked me up at my dorm, and we went to a party at a mansion that was owned by the parents of a friend of his. The third-story party room overlooked a small pond. It was snowing. Alex stood behind me at the window. We watched skaters carving figure eights on the ice. The heat between us was so intense, it could have melted the icicles that hung from the eaves.

Between that day in the cafeteria and the night of the party, we went from "Who's that?" to "This is it." We spent every spare minute together after that.

One day, we went to the music lounge to listen to jazz. As we sat side by side, we talked about what our dream house would look like and drew a sketch of it on a napkin. Ten years later, we built a modified version of that house

By the end of the semester, madly in love, we dreamed of going to California. When we discovered we'd made an early start on having a family, you'd think that might have presented a problem, but it simply provided us an incentive to follow our dream. We were both in our junior year, didn't have, as my mother used to say, a pot to piss in or a window to throw it out of, but we never let things like that deter us.

We married in November and, trailing a Just Married sign behind our red Volkswagen, set out for California. We set up housekeeping in Laguna Beach. Alex got a job as a parts manager at a foreign-car dealership in town, and I stayed home in our little apartment on Blue Bird Canyon. When I went into labor, we made it to the hospital just in time for the doctor to skid into the delivery room and make a miracle catch of our beautiful, supercharged son, Gregor.

A year later, we qualified as California residents, which meant we were eligible for in-state tuition. Alex applied to Berkeley and was accepted. He had two more years to get his bachelor's and another year for his master's degree. We packed up the VW and arrived in Berkeley just in time to witness the beginning of the revolution.

I'm old now, 75 on my last birthday, but, when I hear The Mamas' & The Papas' "California Dreamin'," I'm back in Berkeley. Almost as soon as we arrived, Alex grew a beard and long hair. I tried to ditch my bra, but Mother Nature had generously endowed me, and I wasn't comfortable with "the girls" going freestyle, so I settled on wearing long cotton dresses and going barefoot.

On the weekends, we joined other hippie families in Provo Park to hear Country Joe and the Fish, and The Loading Zone play—for free. They sang anti-war songs and rhapsodized about peace and freedom. Although weed was as common as...well... weed, somehow, I knew my neurology wasn't wired to handle anything stronger. And, besides, somebody had to watch Gregor who, unless we had him by the hand, was fearless and loved "exploring." I never did resort to tying him to a clothesline, but, truth be told, I can't say I wasn't tempted.

Although the Peace and Freedom movement was boiling, the Black Panther Party was seething, and the End the War movement was raging, we still needed to buy diapers and groceries and pay the rent. Alex had a student placement job on campus, but money was tight. I took an exam to qualify as a youth worker at a massive, youth facility located just outside the Bay area. I've always been a good test taker, so I passed with high marks and, armed with recommendations from Manida Street juvie in NYC, getting the job was the easy part. Working the job was another story.

The treatment center combined several types of facilities on one massive campus, and I was often shifted from one unit to another, depending on need. One day, I might be working in the girls' juvenile hall; the next day, I might do three days in the boys' side of the center; on another day, I might be working in the building dedicated to caring for little kids who were victims of abuse or neglect. Sometimes, I spent a week working in the Girls' Residence, which was like a long-term foster home for teen girls.

One night, I was on intake duty at Receiving which meant we were in charge of booking-in girls who'd been detained or arrested. About 11:30 p.m., the police buzzed the outer door. I let in the officer, who was accompanied by a young girl, maybe fourteen or fifteen. Barefooted, her hair and clothes were filthy. She was laughing and crying and mumbling incoherently. The officer told me she'd been cleared at the hospital ER, so we were bound to take her. He handed me the booking folder.

"The doctor said she was on LSD, so let her sleep it off. She'll be fine in the morning." He gave me an enigmatic smile and left.

The girl blew him kisses. I took a minute to read the info in the folder; her name was Olivia.

When I saw the name of her parents, I almost dropped the file. Her father was a Hollywood headline actor, and yet here was his daughter, filthy dirty and zonked out of her mind. I called my supervisor, and we agreed we'd keep her in the observation room overnight with a fifteen-minute watch. The supervisor would try to contact Olivia's parents. I was the watch person for the rest of that shift. Every time I looked through the observation window, Olivia was either sobbing or was curled in a fetal position, clearly in the grip of terrifying emotions and visions. I felt for her and tried to go into the observation room to comfort her, but the supervisor put the kibosh on my efforts.

"Hey," she said, "if the kid was dumb enough to take that stuff, let her take her medicine. Besides, if she goes off and assaults you, there'll be a ration of shit to deal with."

I needed the job. I have few regrets, but I've always felt bad I didn't at least try to help the kid calm down. I'd seen a few folks on a bad trip; sometimes, all they needed was someone calm to reassure them that this would pass.

The next morning, the family attorney flew in and took the kid in hand. She left juvie, unscathed except for whatever residuals she might suffer from the bad trip. She was lucky. Later in my career, I saw several adults who'd come out to California for what was called the Summer of Love. They took their first hit of LSD, and it triggered some sort of latent psychosis or schizophrenic-like state from which they never returned.

The saddest kids I saw were runaways. Of the dozens of young girls booked into juvie, many had fled abusive homes. They came to California seeking the groovy life and ended up on the streets; hungry, dirty, lost—prey to which ever guy promised them a night's sleep and good drugs. A few of the girls were just acting out of basic teenage rebellion and, once they'd had a taste of street life, were anxious to contact their parents and go back home to Indiana or Pennsylvania. Sadly, more often than not, the girls who'd fled abusive homes got stuck in a cycle of prostitution and drug abuse that they likely never did get out of.

I liked the work, the kids, and most of my co-workers, but my schedule was grueling. For one thing, I was working the three-to-eleven afternoon shift. The facility was about 40 minutes away from Berkeley, so I'd get Gregor ready for the babysitter, leave for work around 2:00 p.m., arrive about 15 minutes before shift time and then work (with a 30-minute break for dinner) until 11:00 p.m., do a quick briefing with the overnight staff members, get in the car, drive home, arrive about midnight, do what I needed to do to get ready for the next day, fall into bed around 1:00 a.m., get up at 6:00 a.m., fix breakfast for Alex and Gregor, do laundry, get groceries, wet my parched lips, then start the routine over again. After a year of that, I was zombified and so tired it was all I could do just to stay awake. Many years later, my workaholism would almost kill me.

We spent three years in Berkeley. Alex graduated *summa cum laude* and received his master's degree. He was offered a job in Connecticut, and, since both of our extended families were on the East Coast, we packed up the VW and headed back east.

After a cross-country trip in our trusty, red car, Alex, Gregor, and I arrived in Connecticut. I was also carrying a little passenger, born later that year on the first day of spring—our sunshine girl named Samantha, nicknamed Mandy.

We bought a little, old, brick house in the country. Then it was my turn to go back to school. I found an amazing adult degree program through Goddard College in Vermont and resumed my quest to complete my education.

5

BROKENHEARTED

I earned my BA from Goddard College. Located in Vermont, it had a special program for adult learners, and they were willing to count my prior college credits toward my degree. I graduated with my bachelor's and was then accepted into the University of Connecticut's School of Social Work. Two years later, I graduated with my Master of Social Work degree.

Although I'd intended to begin my career, I didn't want to be tied down to a nine-to-five job. After so many hours of school, I really wanted to spend time with my kids. Luckily for me, a friend of mine had a private practice and invited me to join her in running groups. That was the perfect solution. Over the next two years, I began to see a few individual clients and eventually segued into full-time, private practice.

I had a number of gay women visit my practice. Back then, homosexuality was an issue for some of my colleagues, but, maybe because my favorite aunt and my godmother were both gay, accepting someone's sexual orientation was never a problem for me.

During my days in private practice, Paula, a former client, called to ask if I could see a friend of hers. Jane, she said, had been seeing a therapist for over a year for panic attacks but hadn't found any relief and seemed to be getting worse. Working with Jane turned out to be one of the most moving experiences of my professional life.

"I told her you'd really helped me, and, if you didn't think you could help her, you'd be straight with her and tell her where she could find some help."

I never was a Jill of all trades. I was touched that Paula had enough faith to know that, if I felt I wasn't the right "fit" for a client, I'd work hard to make sure he or she got a referral to a good therapeutic match. The next morning, Jane called. We set up an appointment for the end of the week.

I'd just rented a new office and, while I waited for her, I took a minute to brew myself a cup of coffee and admire my new digs. My office was located on the second floor of a bank building, and one whole side of my session room had a bank of windows that overlooked the street. An F.W. Woolworth store was located catty-cornered across from my building, and my new leather chair next to the windows allowed me to see the goings-on in the street below.

On sunny days, I watched for the Chicken Man, a guy who was a part-time resident of the nearby state hospital. Sometimes, when he was out on a day pass, he liked to put on a dress and combat boots and stroll down the street, walking a chicken on a leash. I don't have a clue where he kept the chicken, but his joie de vivre always brightened my day.

When I heard my waiting room door open, I gulped the last sip of coffee and went to meet my new client.

Jane, wearing a plaid shirt and jeans, had pixie-cut, red hair. I was surprised when she told me she was a licensed electrician, because she was tiny and looked like an elf. In our first meeting, Jane was open, talking about her difficult background as the only child of an alcoholic mother.

"My mom used to work as a maid in a motel. I went to trade school so's I could get a good job and she wouldn't have to work so hard cleaning up after nasty people. I paid for her to go to school to get her practical nurse license last year." She sighed heavily. "But she's still cleaning." Jane sounded like the mother of the two.

With no warning, a sheen of sweat appeared on Jane's forehead, and all color drained from her face. She bent forward, clutched her chest, gasping like she was having a heart attack. I was about to dial 911 when she sat up, wiped her forehead, and took a few deep breaths.

"This is the...anxiety..." she whispered. "Wow, that was a bad one."

Although chest pain, sweating, and labored breathing can be signs of a panic attack, my gut told me that what I'd just witnessed wasn't a panic attack. The symptoms came on out of the blue, which isn't all that unusual, but they disappeared almost as quickly. That wasn't so usual. I stored that thought.

"Jane, what did you just do to manage that attack?"

"Well, Sparrow, my other therapist, worked with me on surfing the waves of anxiety and on breathing and visualizing..." She stopped. "And I try to do that, but I still get 'em."

"Those are all good things to do and should have helped by now. What did you do this time to make the symptoms go away so fast?"

"Well...they just stopped."

"Is that how it usually happens? The attack just comes and then goes away?"

"Pretty much."

"Did Sparrow ever see you having an attack?"

"Yeah."

"Did she ever recommend medication to help you through?"

"No. She doesn't believe in drugs."

Jane's answer was becoming more frequent. When I explored the use of medication to help clients through a serious depression or other bio-behavioral issue, they often said the same thing: "I don't believe in drugs." Somewhere along the line, street drugs and medication have been lumped together as "bad." Maybe by those who believe there's a conspiracy by pharmaceutical companies or by the huge wave of folks seeking natural remedies; nothing wrong with that, but their level of misinformation is often massive, and they will defend their natural-way-of-life choices against all cogent arguments that natural doesn't automatically mean healthy.

I once had a client who was a dedicated Natural is Always Better devotee. She also happened to be bipolar and, at the urging of a Swami she met at the health food store, went off her lithium (by the way, a naturally occurring salt) in favor of "natural" Ayurvedic herbs. A week later, she was found wandering stark naked down Main Street, caught up in a manic episode. But that's another story.

To return to the mystery of Jane's panic attacks, I asked if she'd been to a doctor for a check-up.

"No, I don't like doctors, and Sparrow didn't either." She folded her arms across her chest. I got the message.

I explained that, given the swift onset and intensity of her symptoms and that she'd tried to control them for over a year, I wasn't going to be comfortable treating her for anxiety until I knew she had a clean bill of health. I tried to explore why she hated doctors.

"They're just trying to get your money...and put you on drugs."

Her answer sounded like a rote recitation to me. I suspected that might have been partly Sparrow's philosophy, but that didn't alter the fact that Jane didn't trust doctors. Now I was about to ask her, right off the bat, to go do the thing she'd just told me she hated.

"I hear you. A lot of people feel like you do, but sometimes we gotta do things we really don't like."

Jane pursed her lips and looked me in the eye. "Paula said you were a hardass."

"Takes one to know one." That was not an answer in the theoretical book of Approved Therapist Responses. We looked each other in the eye for a second, and then Jane laughed out loud.

I recommended she get a check-up from Cynthia McMahon, a doctor who was a friend of mine and who practiced a moderate form of holistic medicine.

"If she thinks you need any follow-up tests, she'll help you get hooked up with somebody good...okay?"

I wasn't a doctor, and there was no need at that point to worry her any more than she was, but I suspected there was something not right with Jane's heart. I told her to call me to let me know what the outcome was as soon as she'd seen Cynthia, and we'd set up our next appointment so we could start working together.

Two weeks later, Jane called.

"Dr. Cynthia wanted me to see a cardiologist. She got me in to see the guy, and now he wants me to go for an MRI." She sounded stressed.

"Do you have it set up yet?"

"He set it up when I was there. My mom's gonna take me on Friday."

"Will you call me as soon as you know the results?"

I had mixed feelings. On the one hand, maybe my gut had been right; on the other, I didn't want that to be so. I'd have to wait out the weekend before I heard anything. On Monday afternoon, I was just leaving my office when the phone rang. I picked up.

"Pinny?"

I didn't recognize the voice. "Yes."

"Pinny, I'm Natalie, Jane's mother. She told me to call you about the heart test."

"Oh, I'm so glad you called. I'd been waiting to hear."

"They did an MRI, and they said there's something in her chest..." Her voice broke.

My own heart sank. "Did the doctor give you any idea what's going on?"

"They're going to do more tests, and he said he didn't want to borrow trouble. That doesn't sound good, does it?"

"Natalie, I don't know what the doctor is thinking, and who wouldn't worry, but at least someone is trying to find out what's making Jane sick, and that's a good start." I'm a hopemonger, but my answer sounded thin, even to me. "Thanks so much for calling me and letting me know how the test went. When Jane feels up to it, would you have her give me a call?"

"Well, Jane said you were very nice. I hope you can help her. She's all I have."

"Natalie, I have a daughter too, so I understand how precious Jane is. Let's pray for good news."

Jane called on Tuesday. "Um…I had the MRI, and Dr. Stam said he sees something near my heart." Her voice sounded thin and worried.

"What does he want you to do next?"

"More tests, in the hospital."

"Jane, do you want to come in and talk before your next tests?"

She was crying. "Yes…I'm so scared, and my mom is really freaked out."

"Well, who wouldn't be? Have you had any more panic attacks?"

There was silence on the other end then. "He said he doesn't think I'm having panic attacks…he thinks it might be a heart thing."

Shit, is what I thought. What I said was, "Would you and your mom like to come in and talk? It's up to you."

"Yeah, she's a mess, and I gotta figure this out."

I made some schedule adjustments and was able to see Jane and her mom the next day. Natalie was an older version of her daughter; thin and wiry with the same short-cropped, red hair.

After introductions, we sat down in my office. I sat in my chair next to the window, Jane curled up on the loveseat across from my chair, and Natalie sat down at the other end of the loveseat.

"I suggested to Jane that you two might want to have a chance to talk about what's going on with her."

"*What's going on!*" Natalie almost levitated out of her seat. "I told her to stop seeing that quack, but did she listen? *No*! Now there's something wrong with her heart." Natalie swiped her runny nose with her arm then turned toward Jane. "Didn't I tell you to stop seeing the quack? *Didn't I?*" She was sobbing.

I was confused. Did she mean the doctor? I went over to Natalie, squatted down next to her, and handed her a wad of tissues. She wiped her face and blew her nose loudly.

"Nat? What quack? Dr. McMahon?"

"*No.*"

"Dr. Stam?"

She shook her head no, head still down. "Not them…the bird brain." She sounded disgusted.

"She means Sparrow," Jane said.

Truthfully, I'd had a similar thought about Sparrow. How can you see a client for a year, see the symptoms I'd seen, and, after a few months with no improvement, not try to find out what the heck was going on with the client?

I was aware my own anger was carrying me onto thin ice because, like Natalie, I was mad. Jane was facing a serious health issue, because someone who should have known better hadn't taken the time to find out what the problem really was. But my getting angry wasn't going to help Nat and Jane work through their concerns. I stood up and went back to my chair.

"Jane, what do you need from your mom that might help you?"

Jane looked up at me, like a very small child. "Stop saying bad things about Sparrow."

I looked to Natalie, slumped in the corner of the sofa, rhythmically wadding the tissues into a tight ball. My heart went out to her. Here was a hardscrabble mother whose only child was ill and was, in a way, her lifeline. It's only human to find someone to blame, and Sparrow was it.

"Nat? Did you hear what Jane said? Do you think you can help her feel better by laying off comments about Sparrow?"

Mirroring her daughter's demeanor, Nat mumbled, "Never did like the bitch."

I was surprised. I hadn't known that Natalie knew Sparrow personally.

"Oh, you know Sparrow?"

Like a cloud of dark smoke, a thick silence settled over the room. I let it hang in the air for a while then broke the stalemate.

"What's the story on Sparrow?"

Nat sighed. "We dated."

Most of the time during a therapy session, a therapist's internal dialogue is different from what is said out loud. In this case, I was thinking, *Holy cow. Sparrow and Nat were lovers, and now she's blaming her ex-lover, whom she trusted to treat her daughter, for not recognizing Jane's heart trouble. I wonder if she's also blaming herself.*

Jane sneered. "Dated? You guys were together for two years. Sparrow was good to me…every night when you were at the motel…" Jane raised her arms up in a "what the hell" gesture and stopped mid-sentence.

I mentally filled in the unsaid with a variety of bad choices.

"Did Sparrow live with you all?" I asked Jane.

"Sometimes."

I turned to Natalie. "How long ago were you and Sparrow…dating?"

"A long time ago." Nat ran her fingers through her short-cropped hair.

Jane turned toward her mother. "You broke up with her when I was *twelve*."

There was accusation in her voice. Natalie sat silently, compressing the wadded tissues into a tighter ball. Their simmering resentment was coloring the present, and I wasn't sure if it would be better to try to process the Sparrow issue or to focus on the much more critical problem of helping Jane and her mother deal with Jane's pending diagnostic tests that might have life-changing consequences.

I heard a police siren and glanced out the window. Red lights flashing, a patrol car had stopped in front of Woolworth's. I had to make an effort to pull myself away from the window and refocus on the messy situation at hand.

"Look, I understand the issue of Sparrow is a heavy one for both of you, and I don't want to just sweep it under the rug, but it seems like, for right now, what's important is helping each other get through the next round of tests. Can we agree to just put Sparrow on the shelf until we know more?"

Natalie looked up and nodded.

Jane said, "Yeah, okay. So, now what?"

"Well, besides the two of you, who else is in your support system?"

"Well," said Nat, "I got friends at work and my AA sponsor..." Ah, the things you find out when you think you know what you're doing. I was laughing at myself, because you never know what you don't know when you're working with people. Actually, it was one of the things I loved about being a therapist—the surprise factor. As Forrest Gump's mother used to say, "Life is like a box of chocolates—you never know what you're gonna get."

So, I go into a session thinking I'm going to talk to a mother and daughter about pending diagnostic testing of the heart, and I find out my client's mother is a gay, recovering alcoholic whose one-time lover was my client's former therapist. In a strange way, I guess the session was about the diagnosis of heart problems—just not the ones I thought.

The session ended with an agreement that Natalie would call me with results of the next test, and we'd go from there.

Natalie rang the next week with the worst news possible. Jane had a tumor in her chest, near her heart. Between sobs, she told me the doctors said it was so rare they only had limited experience treating it, and they were going to send her to New York City to see a specialist.

Natalie took Jane there to begin aggressive radiation and chemotherapy. Two months later, she called to tell me Jane was very sick but wanted to see me. I went down to the City to visit her.

I felt sick when I walked into her room. Jane's tiny body barely made a bump in the sheet. She'd lost her red hair and looked like a very old baby. Tubes ran out in every direction. She was heavily sedated but smiled wanly when she saw me. I sat down next to her bed.

"I'm gonna die." Her words were a little slurry. "This shit," she pulled down her johnny coat to show me a port implanted to deliver chemo, "is just putting it off." I nodded. Natalie had told me Jane was receiving hospice care.

I reached out to gently hold her hand, frail as a bird's leg. "Jane, I want to thank you. You taught me something really important. I learned from you to pay attention to not only what a person says but also to pay more attention to their physical health. That lesson is a gift." She looked dreamy and drifty but nodded and squeezed my hand.

"God bless and keep you," I said. Tears slid down my cheeks.

Jane mumbled something. I bent down closer to hear.

With a shadow of a smile, she slurred, "I thought you were a hardass."

I sat holding her hand, listening to the street noise floating up from seven stories below. She dozed off. Before I left, I placed my hand on her forehead.

"God bless and keep you, dear Jane, and make His face to shine upon you and give you peace." I wiped my tears and took the elevator down to the lobby. The door slid open. Nat was standing there, wearing an old, brown sweater that was too big. She looked bedraggled, like a war orphan, which, in some sense, was the truth.

"Can I talk to you for a minute?" she asked.

I asked a nurse if there was someplace where we could meet, and she directed me to a room outside the hospital chapel. As soon as the door to the tiny room closed, Natalie burst into tears. "She's gonna die. What am I gonna dooo?" She was sobbing, and there was nothing to do but share her sorrow with my presence. I silently prayed for her and for Jane. After a while, the sobbing grew less intense. Natalie wiped her nose on her sleeve.

"Honest to God, I can't stand it. I can't live without her...what am I gonna dooo?"

There was no answer that would even begin not to sound clichéd, so I stayed quiet and listened to her talk about Jane. After a long while, it seemed as if Natalie had run out of tears.

"Nat, you raised a very special girl, and I know there is nothing you wouldn't do for her. I'm so sorry her journey is coming to a close. I want you to know she's given me a lesson that will be passed on to others who may come to see me. I hope you'll let your sponsor and friends be there for you. Nat, please have someone call me when…"

She nodded.

Three days later

A phone call at 2:00 a.m. is never good news. I picked up.

"She's gone." Natalie sounded exhausted.

"God bless her. Nat, is anyone with you?"

"Kelly, the hospice nurse…and Sparrow."

That woke me up. Sparrow. I quashed any reaction or questions. My feelings about Sparrow at that time were immaterial. In retrospect, people from one's past often appear or are summoned to return to the side of the dying. I hoped that Jane, Natalie, and Sparrow had healed old wounds and that that had brought them a sense of peace.

"Have you made plans for her service?"

"Blake Funeral Home, the viewing is Tuesday." Her voice was devoid of emotion.

"Is someone going to take you back to Connecticut?"

"Sparrow."

"I'm glad you're not alone, Nat."

"I am alone."

My stomach knotted. I thought I understood what she was saying. "Nat, I'll say a prayer for Jane and for you. And I'll see you at the service."

"Okay." She hung up.

I didn't get back to sleep. It was Saturday morning. I went out to the screened porch with a cup of coffee and thought about the strange twists life takes. A girl comes in for panic attacks; three months later, she's dead. I thought about Natalie and what the rest of her journey would be like. I wanted to tell her again: Jane had made a difference and wouldn't be forgotten.

At 9:30 a.m., the phone rang. "Is this Pinny?"

"Yes." I didn't recognize the voice.

"This is Sparrow."

It's hard to render me speechless. It took a second to even process the fact that the mysterious Sparrow was calling me.

"Sparrow?" What in the world…?

"Um…I thought I should call you. Natalie died."

Sparrow was far more upset than I imagined. For some reason, she was calling to tell me about Jane. Maybe I was on some kind of calling list.

"Sparrow, thanks for letting me know about Jane, but Nat called early this morning to tell me."

"No. Jane died yesterday. Natalie had an aneurysm this morning and died."

"*Natalie* died?"

Speechless twice in the space of a minute.

"I went over to take her to the funeral home to pick out Jane's casket, and she didn't answer the door, so I went to the neighbor who had a key, and we found her on the floor of the bathroom.

The ambulance came. She was cold, but they took her to the hospital."

I couldn't help but wonder if Natalie had committed suicide.

"How do they know it was an aneurysm?"

"I don't know. Some doctor at the hospital said she had an aortic aneurysm that burst."

I didn't know what to say or think. Sparrow filled in the silence. "We're going to cancel the viewing for Jane. She would have hated people gawking at her dead body, and she wanted to be cremated anyway, and when they release Natalie to the funeral home, she'll be cremated. We were thinking maybe we could mix the ashes…what do you think?"

"Ah…Sparrow, it sounds like you're taking care of things; did Jane or Natalie have any relatives?"

"Weird…I know…but they didn't have any family that I ever heard of. When we were together, Nat gave me her power of attorney, and, once we were over, neither of us thought to change it. Now I guess I'm the one that has to figure things out. So, about mixing the ashes…"

"Sparrow, you knew them much better than I. Whatever you think they'd want. Are you going to have separate services or just one for both of them?"

"Me and her sponsor figured we'd have one service when everybody can come, and then we'd take their ashes and strew them off Sound Beach. They both loved the beach."

"Sparrow, that sounds just right. When are you having it?"

"Friday, 11 a.m. at Blake's, then we'll caravan to the Sound and, afterwards, meet for dinner at The Lobster Shack. Do you think that's okay?"

I WENT TO THE SERVICE. THE PLACE WAS FILLED WITH A BOUQUET OF beautiful, old, young, laughing, crying women. Through the crowd, Sparrow and I somehow recognized each other.

"Sparrow?"

"Pinny?"

She led me to the front of the room where an exquisite blue cloisonné urn embellished with an image of two butterflies was flanked by pictures of Jane and Natalie.

"It's perfect," I whispered. Head bowed, I silently prayed for them.

I sat in the back of the room and listened to Jane and Nat's friends tell stories about them. Late afternoon sunlight streamed through stained-glass windows, painting the urn with light. At the end, an older woman, wearing a minister's white collar, recited a short poem followed by a blessing.

I trailed the caravan to the beach. The sun was just starting to set. Sparrow carried the urn to the water's edge. I stood on a dune and watched the ashes float over the ocean and settle into the dark blue sea.

I scuffed down the dune and headed home.

———

IRONICALLY, JUST AFTER I'D FINISHED WRITING THE STORY OF JANE and Nat, which happened years ago, I heard that, a day after Carrie Fisher died, her mother, Debbie Reynolds, passed away. I wasn't as surprised as most. Jane and Nat were way ahead of them.

6

THE MAD MILLIONAIRE, M.D.

At five minutes to four on a Thursday afternoon, I was in my office, waiting to meet a new client referred to me by an attorney who'd sent me several other clients seeking help with mental health issues. I heard the waiting room door open then immediately slam shut. The door to my inner office flew open, and a beefy guy blew in, dressed in an expensive but rumpled suit. His hair looked like a mass of gray Brillo. His shirt was untucked and spattered with stains. Eyes darting in panic, he dropped to the floor and crawled on his knees toward the couch. Riveted to my chair, I was, as Brits would say, gobsmacked.

I took a minute to observe the poor man, who appeared to have just escaped from Bedlam. He sat on the floor, back against the couch, twitching like a horse in fly season. His eyes continued to scan the room as if he were being stalked by vipers. *What the hell...is this my four o'clock appointment? Is this Dr. Felix Graves, the guy my attorney friend referred? Is this Dr. Felix Graves, the plastic surgeon? If so, Dr. Graves is clearly in need of intensive care himself.*

He was far too disorganized to carry on a coherent conversation, but it didn't seem like he was a threat, so I decided to just sit quietly until he'd had a chance to scope out the office and settle down a little. He pulled a grubby handkerchief from his pocket and wiped his sweaty face. When he blew his nose, I saw blood on the handkerchief. That gave me more than a little pause. I started to try to put some of the puzzle pieces together based on what I was seeing.

Disheveled, professional man bursts into a private office; he's panic-stricken, hypervigilant, likely paranoid; he's twitchy and has a nose bleed. Aw, geez, is this guy a speed freak? Naw...he's a doctor. I mentally smacked myself on the back of the head. *Doctor, schmoctor...speed is rampant in this city, and doctors are just as prone as the next guy to get hooked. Okay, sister, don't be hasty. Is there any other diagnosis that might explain his behavior? Of course there is, let's say maybe he's bipolar and in the grip of a manic episode. Okay, what else? Maybe he was being chased by men in black...Hmmm.* While I was musing, the guy spoke up.

"Can anybody hear us?"

Okay, check. He's paranoid.

"No." I lowered my voice. "Are you Dr. Graves?"

"Yes, can you close the shades?"

I got up and drew all the window shades.

"Is that better?" I put genuine concern in my voice. The poor guy was really scared. "I see that something has you worried. Are you in a position to tell me what has upset you, or would you rather take a few minutes so we can get the basics sorted out?"

"Look, I don't even know why I'm here. The lawyer said I should come."

"Was that Attorney Shelton? Is he your attorney?"

"Yes." His eyes continued to scan the room. I assumed he was looking for bugging devices. He was itching his arms and face like he had poison ivy, but, by now, I'd pretty much concluded he was on a speed binge.

"I can't tell you...the thing is...what am I gonna do...?" He wasn't asking me that question. It was the cry of a man on the edge of despair.

I reached down and opened the mini fridge by my desk and handed the good doctor a chilled bottle of water. He took it, rubbed the cold bottle against his face, twisted off the cap, and drained it in huge gulps.

"How about we take a few minutes so I can get your basic information?"

"*No!*" His arm shot up. "Don't write anything down."

I was starting to feel a tiny bit worried. He was a big guy, agitated and paranoid. Maybe the better part of valor would be to just walk out the exit door at the other end of the room and call 911. In any case, it was clear I wasn't going to conduct a regular intake interview. So now what? Anyone presenting with the same behaviors of desperation as the doctor might be a candidate for suicide. *Ask now or wait?*

Once he'd drained the water bottle, the doctor seemed a little calmer. He continued to sit on the floor, back against the couch. He pulled out his bloodied handkerchief and once again blew his nose. Nothing ventured...I figured I'd try to find a way to connect with him through his professional side.

"Dr. Graves, I know you've been in my position, where you have to ask a patient a question you know might upset them, but you have to ask it anyway?" He looked at me. For a second, he looked like he was connecting. "Are you thinking about suicide?"

Sometimes, people are afraid to ask someone if they're thinking of suicide, because they fear they may plant the idea, but my experience has been that, if someone isn't suicidal, they'll snort or dismiss the idea out of hand. But if suicidal ideation is lurking, often, not always but often, that person will openly admit that it's occurred to them or that they're thinking about it, and, for some, it's a relief to talk about it. However, that was not the case with Dr. Graves.

"I'm sorry I've bothered you, but I have to go." He levered himself to his knees, stood up, and dashed out the door.

Oddest interview, or non-interview, ever. I felt unsettled about letting the doctor leave in the state he was in, and I was up in the air about what to do, if anything. I decided to call Tim Shelton, the attorney who'd referred the doc, to see if he could, or would, be able to shed some light on the situation. Although it was now almost five o'clock, I got lucky and caught Tim before he'd left the office.

"Tim, it's Pinny. I just finished seeing Dr. Graves." There was a long silence on the other end.

Finally, he asked, "Whaddaya think?"

"I think he's gone off the deep end. He was a mess. What's his story?"

Tim sighed. "I was afraid you were going to ask that. I can't tell you any details, but I was worried."

"Tim, I'm not accusing the doctor of anything, but d'you know if he's ever had any drug problems?"

"God, I wish I could tell you, but..."

"So, what d'you think I should do? Am I under any legal obligation to do anything?"

"Did he make any threats against anybody?"

"Nope, wouldn't even answer basic questions."

"You're in the clear. Did he say anything about anything?"

"Nothing coherent."

"Pinny, I wish I could tell you something...but attorney-client privilege..."

"I understand. But do me a favor, does he have a wife, or do you know anyone you could call or...would you call him? That poor guy is on the edge."

"I'll call the wife, but this is a really sticky situation."

"Well, listen, thanks for the referral. I'm really sorry I wasn't any help to him."

"Pinny, thanks for trying. I'll keep in touch."

Even after I'd talked to Tim, I was worried about letting a client walk away who was in such a state. Although he'd appeared for an appointment, he hadn't given me any personal information, so I wasn't even sure if he qualified as a client. But I couldn't figure out what else, if anything, I could have done.

He was disorganized and paranoid but hadn't made any

threats to me or anyone else. He'd denied or, more accurately, ignored my query about feeling suicidal.

I briefly thought about calling the police but I was pretty sure he wouldn't have met any of the criteria for an arrest. And what about my obligation to maintain confidentiality? I'd called his attorney and alerted him to the situation and had gotten his reassurance that I'd fulfilled my legal obligations, and the attorney told me he'd follow up, but…something wasn't right. I watched the papers for the next month to see if any news emerged about the doc. Over the next months, my worry faded.

The rest of the story

One year later, the newspaper headlines were all about a doctor who'd hired a hitman to kill his partner. It turned out that, about six months after I saw the doctor, his partner was shot during what first appeared to be a botched robbery. After another six months of investigation, the doctor was arrested for murder. News reports revealed the doctor had been deeply enmeshed in drug dealing, and, when he'd gotten in over his head, he'd arranged to have his partner killed for the insurance money. No wonder the doc was twitchy.

7

CRASH AND BURN

After fifteen years in private practice, I had two offices and a large client load. I was commuting between my home office and my office in New Haven and frequently stayed up late to catch up on paperwork. Although I had several colleagues I used for backup, I made it my practice to personally answer my clients' phone calls. I didn't recognize the toll the work was taking on me until I came down with viral meningitis, an inflammation of the dura around the brain. Shortly after that, I contracted pericarditis, which is, ironically, a virally caused inflammation of the sack around the heart—no metaphor there, folks. Like many of us in the helping professions, I hadn't paid much attention to taking care of myself. After spending so many years sitting in a beige room listening to an unending litany of pain, I was burned out.

The cardiologist and the neurologist agreed that stress had compromised my immune system. The cardiologist ordered mandatory bed rest and medication until the pericarditis cleared. It was the first time in a very long time I'd been forced to just sit down (because lying down when one has pericarditis is most uncomfortable) and face the fact that work had become my drug of choice.

Early on in life, I'd vowed I wouldn't become alcoholic. My dad's alcoholism had been part of the reason for the divorce from my mother, and his drinking had caused me deep and enduring pain. Believing I could outsmart genetics and outrun the early influences of nurture, I'd adopted an alcohol-free lifestyle and smugly thought the whole issue of addiction was therefore handled. But all I'd done was to sidestep alcoholism and substitute workaholism.

Once again, I sought therapy and, at the recommendation of my therapist, I entered a special program, run at that time by the Hazelden Foundation. It was designed especially for therapists, for issues specific to our profession. It was there I began to understand that, for me, work was an addiction. At the end of the program, I came to see it was time for me to step back and reassess if I wanted to spend the rest of my life sitting in a beige room and maybe not live a very long life at all. By then, our children were both launched into the world, and, over the next three months, Alex and I took time together to plan how we wanted to live the rest of our lives.

Because both of us are planners, and Alex was a trainer in systems management at that time, together we mapped out a life-planning program, just for ourselves.

In preparation for our personal life plan workshop, we brainstormed a series of questions to ask ourselves. Questions like: Where do I want to live? What kind of work would I want to do? What kind of activities do I enjoy? What kinds of friends do I want? What are my spiritual needs? And many more.

We then made a reservation at a residence-type motel for the weekend. The suite had a living room, kitchen, and separate bedroom. We brought with us two spiral-bound notebooks, a large pad of paper plus the workshop easel Alex used in his training, and a roll of masking tape.

We checked in and went out to dinner. The next morning, each of us wrote down into our spiral notebook the questions we'd prepared then went to separate rooms and began to write. There were no rules about writing. We could include any wild idea that might occur to us. Two hours later, we came up for air. After lunch, we swapped notebooks then took time to read what the other had written.

We were amazed to find that each of us had separately wanted to move to Florida; we'd been vacationing there for years. Although we'd built a solar house, the Connecticut winters were long and grim, and we loved the sun. Alex taped large tear sheets to the walls and began to write down our various hopes, dreams, and aspirations. We set goals and timelines for each thing we needed to do to begin our new life in Florida. By the end of that weekend, we had the outlines of a bold, new chapter in our lives.

Although we thought we'd covered all our bases, we made two critical mistakes. First, we decided to leave for Florida while our house was on the market. Second, Alex accepted a job offer from a close relative who was initiating a development project in Florida.

Long, painful story short—right after we left, a housing crash began, and our house sat vacant on the market for eighteen months. This meant we were paying rent on a Florida condo and the mortgage on our Connecticut house. And, as it turned out, the relative with the development project was a bona fide con artist who swindled us out of our life savings. As this person was a relative, we hadn't thought signing an employment contract was necessary. Word to the wise: Always. Get. Everything. In. Writing.

So, there we were—shipwrecked upon the rocks of bad judgment. What to do? We did what we've always done. Licked our wounds for a few days then picked up metaphorical shovels and started digging. In a short time, we got our real estate licenses and went to work selling houses.

It turned out I was pretty good at it. I'd had years of figuring out what people were thinking and feeling and was able to transfer those skills into selling. Alex got a job selling commercial real estate. Slowly, like two phoenix birds with singed feathers, we began to rise. The Connecticut house finally sold, and we bought a villa overlooking a golf course.

We joined a church and sang in the choir. Luckily for us, our choir director was also the music director for a massive concert venue, and we had the fun of singing there as backup for Neil Sedaka and several other famous "golden oldies." We made good friends and started to rebuild a little of the financial cushion we'd lost. For five years, I sang, played golf, sold fancy real estate, and had time to reflect on how losing everything had brought me to a place that was filled with peace, fun, and good health.

And then, one morning, as I sat on the patio reading the paper, I saw an ad: "Palmetto Behavioral Health Clinic—Clinician Needed." I was ambivalent about leaving real estate. On the one hand, it often brought big paychecks. On the other, our livelihood was frequently dependent on someone deciding they needed a million-dollar house and on the deal closing before the next batch of bills arrived.

In the preceding five years, I'd learned a lot about how to take care of myself, and the prospect of having a nine-to-five job that had a steady and predictable income plus health benefits loomed large. What could it hurt to go see? I called and made an appointment for an interview.

I was hired provisionally, pending a check of my CV. Soon, I was once again immersed in a fascinating world I thought I'd left behind. Forrest Gump's mother was right once more: life as a clinician at a public mental health clinic is like a box of chocolates—you never know what you're going to get. It's one of the things I loved. I could never guess who would come through my door, but each person was a blessing to me and gave me the honor of sharing a part of their life's journey with them.

8

I SPY

One of the first clients I had at the Palmetto Behavioral Health Clinic was also one of the most unusual.

The intake sheet was almost blank. Other than name, birth date, address, and age—56—there was nothing to give me a clue about my next client, Winifred Small. Her appointment was at 10:00 a.m. I called Peg, the intake worker.

"Peg? Listen, I'm looking at the intake sheet for Winifred Small, and there's no info on it."

"Yeah, well, here's the deal...that's all she'd give me."

Peg was one of the best screeners I've met. Her way of coaxing information out of the most guarded clients made her a great asset to the clinic.

"I tried everything to get her to talk to me, but all she'd say was, and I quote, 'I am not at liberty to reveal the nature of my issue,' end quote."

"Okay. If you couldn't get her to talk, I imagine the assessment is going to be interesting."

"Good luck. I'll buzz you when she gets here."

A few minutes later, the phone rang. Sotto voce, Peg said, "She's heeere."

There were only two people in the waiting room: a guy with a full sleeve of tattoos and a tall woman wearing a gray pantsuit and sensible shoes. I went over to her, leaned down, and in a voice barely above a whisper, said, "Ms. Small, I'm Pinny Bugaeff. Let's go to my office."

Ms. Small stood up. I guessed she was maybe six foot two inches in flats. I pushed open my office door and stepped back to usher her in. She halted on the threshold. The image that came to mind was of a giraffe standing at the edge of a clearing, searching for a lurking leopard.

Winifred stepped into the office and sat down in the chair furthest from my desk. She was more than a little wary and, if that was so, she must be sitting on something really disturbing, because it's rare for truly paranoid people to voluntarily come into therapy. Since she was dressed more formally than my usual casual Florida client, I chose to use formal language.

"Ms. Small, I noticed you gave our intake worker only a minimum of personal information, and I want you to know I think it's prudent to take the time to assess the situation before one reveals too much."

For people who have a high degree of suspicion, trust is a tricky issue. When a client appeared to be guarded, I usually tried to embed some message that affirmed their right to keep their issue to themselves. That may sound paradoxical, but one goal of therapy is to identify the issues causing the pain, and I felt like it actually helped patients feel a little safer to reassure them they didn't have to reveal themselves without taking time to feel more comfortable.

Winifred settled back in her chair and scanned the office. I pushed her paperwork away and put my pen down, a nonverbal signal that I wasn't taking notes. I decided to start with very simple questions.

"Ms. Small, how long have you lived in Florida?"

"Five years."

"Do you have family in Florida?"

"No."

Her lips pressed together, and she grimaced, a micro-movement that sometimes signals disgust. She tried to maintain her impassive demeanor, but her unconscious reaction might indicate what she thought about her relatives or family.

I filed that reaction away and moved to another subject. "Do you work?"

"Yes."

"How would you feel about telling me what you do?"

"I am a secretary."

I hadn't asked her what she did. I'd asked her how she would feel about telling me what she did. Her answer about her job didn't seem to make her uneasy, so I pushed a little further.

"And you work for...?"

"I work for the County Water Commission."

"Do you have any hobbies?" I was trying to stay on neutral ground until I saw some reduction in Ms. Small's level of tension, but her posture was still rigid and her answers terse.

"I volunteer at the church, and I play Yahtzee on Tuesday nights."

My "make haste slowly" mantra was quickly starting to disappear under my "it's almost 10:30 and I've spent half an hour finding out that the church lady is a secretary" reality. But I wasn't any closer to finding out why Winifred was seeking help. What else did I know? She played Yahtzee, so she must have at least a few friends. Her hygiene and grooming were good, and her speech, although sparse, wasn't bizarre. She'd reported some elements of a normal life but was very guarded—so what was going on?

I wondered if her paranoia might just be a deeply shameful thought that she was too embarrassed to voice. Maybe something sexual?

I was struggling until I heard the voice of the old psychiatrist who had mentored me. "When all else fails, better to ask than to speculate." I was aware that now *I* was the one hearing voices.

"Ms. Small, can you give me an idea what it is that made you decide to come to the clinic?"

Brow wrinkled, she frowned like she was displeased that, somehow, I'd failed to intuit her unspoken issue. She sat peering at me through her bifocals. Nothing. I tried once more.

"Before you made this appointment to talk to me, what kind of things did you try in order to deal with your issue?"

"I prayed."

"Did you receive divine guidance?"

"Why do you think I'm here?"

I was flummoxed. "God told you to come to the clinic?"

"God does not speak to me directly." Her tone of voice seemed to indicate that her assessment of me was correct. I was slow.

"I prayed about this matter, and the next morning, when I opened the newspaper, there was an article about the clinic."

She continued to peer at me. I thought she might be trying to see if I understood the connection between praying for something and the newspaper article. I nodded as if I'd immediately made the connection and fell back into therapy-speak.

"I see."

I felt sad I wasn't helping Ms. Small feel safer, because it was becoming clear she wasn't going to divulge whatever it was that had driven her into therapy. So, I sent up my own *God, please help* prayer. While waiting for rescue, I decided to try one more thing.

"I think it must have taken a lot of courage to come in today," I said, "and you have every right to keep whatever is bothering you to yourself, but how do you think you'll feel if you leave today, still carrying the same burden you brought in with you?"

She sat up in her chair and stared at me. "I've carried it this long, what's another day, or week, or year?" She sounded sour and defeated. She pursed her lips.

"And yet you came here with a little prompting from God. I remember a verse from Sunday school. I think it was in Matthew... 'Come to me, all you who are weary and burdened, and I will give you rest.' I have to wonder if maybe you were led to come here because He wants you to feel better by sharing your burden."

She maintained her rigid posture and continued to stare at me.

"For sure I don't know the mind of God, and if you think you'll feel better leaving with what brought you here, I will understand. But it just occurred to me that you don't have to tell me anything. How do you think you would feel if you wrote down your burden? You could write it on a piece of paper, and, to show God you were an obedient servant, we could take it outside and burn it. He would then receive your burden and maybe you'll…" I left off the end of the sentence and hoped she might mentally fill in the blank with "…feel better."

I had no compunction about bringing in a "higher authority" when the occasion called for it. And, in truth, I did believe God was with me and did, sometimes, bless me with divine inspiration. I was not a Christian Therapist per se—a therapist who provides therapy based on Christian principles as elucidated in the Bible. I am, however, a believer in the power and presence of a God who will always provide what I need but, there's a kicker, in His own time. In any case, while Ms. Small appeared to be thinking about my proposal, I tore my shopping list off the pad and pushed the pad toward her, along with the pen.

She reached for them and scribbled something. She bore down so hard on the paper, it looked like she might drill right through. She tore off the page, folded it in fourths and then into eighths. I stood and signaled her to follow me. I had one of the few offices that had a door to an outside patio. On the way out, I grabbed the metal wastebasket.

It was warm outside and humid. A light breeze windmilled the palm fronds, and two white egrets stalked the edge of the property. I glanced to see that no one else was around. Back then, I still smoked, and my Bic was always with me, so I pulled my lighter from my pocket and looked at Ms. Small. Her head was swiveling on her neck like she was watching for that leopard to burst out of the trees and tear her to shreds. I placed the wastebasket at the edge of the patio.

"Do you want to say anything?"

She shook her head no.

"Do you mind if I say something?"

"No."

I didn't know if she meant, no, don't say anything, or no, I don't mind if you say something. I decided to interpret it as the latter.

"Well, God, here is a burden that Your faithful servant Winifred is bringing to You. We hope You will receive it and grant her some peace."

I reached into the basket and removed the few pieces of paper already in it then nodded at Winifred to drop her burden into the wastebasket. She squeezed the tightly folded missive between her fingers then dropped it into the basket. I tore up the papers in my hand, bundled them into a loose nest, dropped them on top of The Burden, then bent down and flicked my Bic. The paper flared, black wisps of carbon wafting upward. The tight, yellow bundle unfurled in the flames. An edge caught fire, and the note was quickly consumed. Once the fire was out, I picked up the wastebasket and tossed the ashes into the wind.

Winifred followed me back into the office. "Ms. Small? I hope you will come back to see me at least one more time so we can see how you're feeling. Will you come back next week?"

She nodded. "I will."

Her demeanor hadn't really changed. She picked up her purse. I led the way down the hall to the waiting room. We stopped at Peg's desk.

"Ms. Small would like to make an appointment for next week."

I left Ms. Small at the desk with Peg and, back in my office, breathed a silent thank you to God for His guidance then sat back down at my desk, turned the pad around, picked up the pen, and began to lightly scribble over the impressions of the words so deeply etched into the paper. When I saw what Winifred had written, I was stunned:

> THE CIA IS WATCHING ME THROUGH MY IUD.

No wonder Winifred was reticent. Her note indicated she was possibly delusional, and her level of paranoia was palpable. But, on second thought, just because the idea was implausible didn't mean it was impossible...did it? The government does have a history of doing some very shady experiments on human subjects. LSD was given to unsuspecting military volunteer subjects in the '60s. Hmmm...I laughed at myself. *Now who's paranoid?*

In any case, Winifred was clearly suffering. I made a mental note to make sure Peg called to remind her of her next appointment and to schedule a psychiatric evaluation when Winifred returned.

The next day, I woke up and glanced out my bedroom window. A great blue heron stood motionless, apparently tracking a bit of tasty prey. Somehow, he reminded me of Winifred Small. I sat up in bed and smacked myself in the forehead. Winifred was well beyond child-bearing age; why was she wearing an IUD? I made a mental note to ask if she showed up for her next appointment then caught myself. She hadn't told me what her secret issue was. I'd sussed it out by scribbling over the impression she left on the note pad.

Winifred did return for her appointment with me and seemed a little less guarded. But I made a decision. There are times when it's better to back out of a situation gracefully rather than risk stumbling into a well-sealed area, releasing an unknown number of toxic fears or memories that could, ultimately, lead to serious consequences in a relatively stable life.

Winifred had some deeply hidden and complex reasoning that had to do with maintaining an IUD, even though she was past child-bearing years and in spite of the fact that the CIA might be eavesdropping on her Yahtzee games.

She appeared right on time for her follow-up session.

"How are you feeling since our last meeting?" I asked, not indicating in any way that I'd been privy to her secret. Truthfully, I felt a little guilty about my snooping.

Winifred stared at me for a second. "Well…" She paused. "I am going to speak to my doctor."

I let her answer hang for a minute. Winifred didn't seem to be any more anxious about the IUD-CIA issue than when I'd seen her previously, and I wondered if just maybe the burning of the burden ritual had served to somehow allay some of her fear. Maybe, maybe not. In any case, I reassured her that, if at any time she wanted to return, my door would be open.

The rest of the story

Some may question my use of the burning ritual in the context of traditional therapeutic practice. It's not something I would use on a regular basis, but, for many people, talking therapy and self-revelation are painful and disturbing processes, especially for someone who's already suspicious or paranoid. Therapy isn't a science. Although there are some schools of treatment that use algorithms in treatment planning, I'm old school. My mantra is to give hope and comfort, share knowledge, do no harm, join the journey. To my way of thinking, there is no one-size-fits-all brand of therapy, but it's our responsibility, if we are to be honored to join others in their quest, to have a wide variety of therapeutic tools in our armamentarium. And, occasionally, the use of a ritual —like maybe burned offerings—is therapeutic.

9

LOVE STORY

Session One

The clinical intake sheet for Sam Hoag read: Date of Birth: 4-7-1934, Everglades City. Occupation: Oysterman. Married 40+ yrs. Wife's name: Clementine. Presenting problem: Client referred by his doctor for depression.

I walked into the waiting room, and a ripe combo of BO, fish, and alcohol wafted toward me. The other clients were standing against the wall rather than sit next to the guy wearing a Greek fisherman's cap. I made an educated guess and went over to him.

"Mr. Hoag?" He sat staring at the floor.

I bent closer to him. "Mr. Hoag? I'm Pinny Bugaeff, the social worker."

He offered me a limp handshake. Despite the stink, my heart went out to him. Poor guy looked like a basset hound wearing a hat. Luckily for me, a long-ago bout of flu had robbed me of most of my sense of smell.

"Sam, let's go to my office."

When he stood up, the plaid Bermuda shorts he wore hung precariously below his belly. I hoped friction would be enough to keep them there. Once in my office, Sam waddled over to the wing chair and plopped down. The smell of old booze hung in the air.

Guys like Sam don't go to therapy. The last thing in the world a man like him would do is to wake up some morning and announce to his wife, "I'm feeling depressed; perhaps I'll schedule a little therapy." On the contrary, I imagined that Sam probably adhered to two primary Swamp Cracker values: Never, ever, tell a stranger anything. And never let anybody think you're "mental."

"Sam, you don't have to tell me if you don't want to, but whose idea was it for you to come here?"

"Wasn't mine."

"So, you didn't want to come to the clinic, but somebody made you?"

"Yep."

You can pry open an oyster's shell or immerse them in gently simmering water.

"Sam, what's it like being an oyster fisherman?"

"It's fuckin' hard." Sam had a lateral lisp. When he spoke, he sounded just like Sylvester the cat. "The fuckin' gov'mint has closed down all the oyster beds. Before that, I had a good business. You ask anybody. I worked every damn day of my life. But the hell with the gov'mint. I'm catchin' 'em anyway. God put those oysters there for catchin' and eatin'."

Sam was angry, but at least he was talking.

"Wasn't for the damned gov'mint, my boy…" Sam stopped mid-sentence. His eyes filled with tears.

"What happened to your boy?"

"He's dead."

I waited to see if he'd tell me more, but he'd retreated behind a thousand-yard stare.

Given this was the first time he'd dipped a toe into therapy, it might be too much, too soon to stir up such deep powerlessness and grief in an already fragile guy. I opted to switch topics.

"Let me just tell you what I know about you, Sam. You're 59 years old. You've lived in the Glades your whole life.

You're an oysterman, and you've been married for 40 years. The government is messing up your business. And you lost a son."

He nodded.

"Can you tell me why you think your doctor suggested you come to therapy?"

"The missus said she wouldn't 'do it' 'til I went to see him."

I nodded.

Dirty, depressed, and drinking, carrying a long list of grievances, and now his wife had cut him off. I decided to do a risk assessment for suicide.

"Sam, I'm going to have to ask you a bunch of questions. Some of them might sound crazy, but I really want to help you, so I'll try to go as quick as I can. Okay?"

He nodded again.

"Sam, do you know what day it is?"

He sat up straighter in the chair and looked at me like I was crazy. "It's Tuesday."

"Who's the president of the United States?"

Sam leaned forward and got louder. "I ain't stupid, ya know…Clinton."

"Right. I know you're plenty smart, Sam, and some of these questions are dumb. I'll try to hurry things up. Sam, do you ever hear voices…but can't see the person who's talking?"

He hesitated for a second. "Yes, I do."

That got my attention. Hearing voices is a serious symptom. Was he hearing random voices or, worse, command hallucinations, like maybe, "The devil is telling me to kill my neighbor."

"When do you hear the voices?"

He sat back and smirked. "When I listen to the radio."

I laughed. Maybe he was joking, but there's a certain type of psychosis that involves the belief that people on the radio or TV are speaking personally to the listener, maybe giving them instructions to harm themselves or others. I couldn't let Sam joke his way out of a possible serious symptom.

"Do you think the voice on the radio is sending you any personal messages?"

"Yes. I do." He nodded several times.

My heart sank. "What are they telling you?"

He looked up at me from under the brim of his cap. "Drink Budweiser." He snorted, laughed, and slapped the desk.

Sam was telling me he'd play my stupid therapy game, but he wasn't dumb. I started feeling a little better, because Sam still had a sense of humor.

"Just a few more questions, okay? Sam, some people who've gone through a lot of bad stuff, like you have, think about killing themselves, or think maybe everyone would be better off without them. Have you ever thought about killing yourself?"

"Naw, but…"

"But?"

He put his hands on the edge of my desk, leaned toward me, and stood up. "I'd like to kill the goddamned sonsabitches that took Billy."

Oh crap. He's not suicidal, he's homicidal.

"So, who would that be?" I had to make a conscious effort to relax. I took a long breath and exhaled slowly. Sam was a powder keg. He turned around and stomped over to the sliding glass door. I was afraid for a second he was just going to march outside and leave. A flock of white ibis landed on the lawn. Way above the palm trees, the sky was filled with puffy, marshmallow clouds. Outside was paradise. Sam's back was to me when he answered my question.

"F--kin' Game Warden Ralph Stiers for one and f--kin' Judge Crampton for another."

I had to find out if the men on his mental hit list were in immediate danger.

"Are they still around?" I asked.

Sam whirled around. His face was almost purple. He looked like he was on the verge of apoplexy. He marched back toward my desk, yelling, "The warden, Stiers, got a *pro-mo-tion*. They sent him to somewhere up north. The f--kin' judge retired."

I was getting more concerned by the minute. I forced myself to sit back and unclench my shoulders. I took a second to glance out the sliding glass door and wished I was outside. Sam flopped back down in the chair.

"Do you know Mr. Stiers' address?"

"*No*, I ain't got the address, but I could get it if I wanted."

"If you wanted to, what would you do to them?"

Sam leaned toward me, placed his clenched fists on the desk, and whispered through clenched teeth.

"I'd blow their asses up...the whole damn rats' nest of 'em."

I was listening closely. His lisp and the intensity of his murmured words made it difficult to catch what he was telling me.

"Sam, do you have any explosives or maybe a friend that could get them for you?"

"No. But I could if I wanted."

"Sam, how many guns do you have?"

He stopped ranting. Looking like a wily, old swamp fox, he glared at me. "How come you want to know how many guns I got?"

"Because I'm concerned that, sometime, you might be having a bad day and—"

He interrupted. "I ain't gonna kill 'em, if that's what yer thinkin'."

"Well...if you *were* thinking about it, have you made any plans about how you'd go after them?"

"Plenty." He stared at me then pulled the bill of his cap down so I couldn't really see his face.

I was getting more worried by the minute. Was I getting into Tarasoff territory? I groaned inwardly.

In 1973, a male student at the University of California, Berkeley, reported to a California psychologist that he'd thought of killing a girl—Tatiana Tarasoff—whom he was obsessed with. Although the psychologist alerted the campus police to the possible danger, after they questioned the student, they just warned him to stay away from the girl. He subsequently killed her.

The university was sued by the girl's parents. The outcome of that suit and a subsequent action established that psychotherapists have both a Duty to Warn and a Duty to Protect potential victims of violence. Duty to Protect means that, when a therapist believes their patient presents a serious danger to another, the therapist must use reasonable care to protect the intended victim against danger, which means informing the intended victim and the police and taking other steps to protect the intended victim.

A potential tsunami of events was building; a grieving father, drinking alcoholically, nursing a grudge against a judge and a game warden, had access to guns and admitted to entertaining thoughts of revenge. For sure, I was going to have to talk to my supervisor. But now I had to try and suss out what plans Sam had made to possibly kill a judge and a game warden.

"Like what kind of plans?"

He leaned toward me and said, "Shove a stick of dynamite up their ass."

Okay. I exhaled. Dynamite up the ass—not exactly a viable plan.

"What else?"

He looked disgusted. "That ain't bad enough?"

I stayed quiet.

"What? You think I won't?" He lifted his pugnacious jaw and squinted at me.

"I don't know; that's why I'm asking you all these questions. Are there any reasons why you might decide not to blow up those guys?"

He stared at the floor. "I can't leave Clemmie and…" He stopped.

"Anyone else who might feel bad if you did something like that?"

"Billy Two." He held up two fingers.

"Who's Billy Two?"

"My grandson." He looked up at me from under the bill of his cap, and I saw tears in his eyes.

"How old is Billy Two?"

"He's seven."

"Where does he live?"

"He's my daughter's boy. They live up in Apalachicola. She named him after her brother."

I was on the fence. Although Sam had passing thoughts of suicide and homicide, he didn't have specific plans. His demeanor indicated that shoving a stick of dynamite up the judge's ass wasn't actually a viable plot. He still had a few shreds of humor left, and he loved his wife and grandson and didn't want to do anything that would cause them pain. Those factors were fairly strong elements of protection that Sam wasn't an immediate danger to himself or others, but his drinking and his access to guns made the situation tricky.

I was pretty sure there wasn't enough to have him Baker Acted—involuntarily institutionalized and examined—but asking him to sign a Contract for Safety might send him out of the office. I didn't really have a choice. Although the idea that having someone who is potentially suicidal or homicidal sign a promise they wouldn't harm themselves or others gave me little reassurance, it was one of the few viable tools I had at that moment.

"Okay. Sam, I think you're a man of your word. Are you willing to promise me you're not going to kill yourself or anyone else? Are you willing to tell Clemmie or call the clinic or 911 if you feel like hurting yourself or the game warden or the judge?"

Sighing, he bowed his head and nodded. "Ah ain't gonna do nuthin'."

I believed him but was still going to keep close tabs on him.

Handing him the pen, I slid the one-page Safety Contract across the desk for him to sign. He scribbled a signature on it then shoved it back across the desk. I gave him a copy and kept one.

"Just a few more questions. Sam, you've lived a long time, doing just fine on your own. So, tell me again, what made you decide to come to the clinic?"

He bent over from the waist and buried his face in his hands. "Clemmie said if I didn't come here, she'd leave me."

"Why do you think she said that?"

"She said I was a miserable son of a bitch and, if I didn't go and get some kind of counseling, she'd go live with our daughter up in Apalachicola."

"Sam, you were a good guy to come in here. But when a client comes in for their first appointment, if they're married, I always want to talk to their husband or wife. You said your wife thinks you're an SOB, but there are two sides to every story. Do you think she'd come in?"

Sam sat up straight. "You want Clemmie to come to counseling? *Shit*, yes. She thinks it's all my fault."

"Will you come back with her?"

"Shit, yes."

"How about tomorrow at two o'clock?" I wanted to get his wife in as soon as possible so I could get a better sense of a potentially dangerous situation. I wrote out an appointment card for him. Later on, I'd call and make sure his wife would come in for a joint session. Sam stood up to leave.

"Sam, you promised you'd call if you start to feel bad, right?"

"I signed the paper, didn't I?"

"Okay then. I'll call Clemmie and see you both tomorrow."

Session Two

Slumped in an untidy heap, Sam was sitting in the waiting room next to a bone-thin woman I assumed was Clemmie. She wore a pale blue, polyester pantsuit and was clutching an alligator bag on her lap. The bag was actually *made* from a baby alligator. The purse part was the 'gator body, and the closure flap was made from the baby 'gator's head.

"Hi, Sam. Mrs. Hoag?" I reached out to shake her hand. "I'm Pinny, the social worker."

She gave my hand one short pump but remained silent.

"Let's go back to my office."

Sam levered himself out of his chair. Clemmie unfolded with the grace of an ironing board. Once in my office, Sam threw himself into the wing chair. I pulled up a chair for Clemmie. Sam's aroma seemed less powerful. Maybe he'd bathed, or maybe that was just my poor sense of smell.

I smiled at Clemmie. "Mrs. Hoag? Please call me Pinny."

I waited for a reciprocal affirmation from Clemmie, but it wasn't forthcoming.

"When we spoke on the phone, I told you I'd like you to come in with Sam because I think it's helpful, when a couple has difficulty, to listen to both sides of the story."

Clemmie said, "Ah ain't the one with the problem." She pursed her lips and stared at Sam. When she did that, it reminded me of what Uncle Clyde used to say about his mother-in-law: "That woman is so prissy, when she puckers up her mouth, it looks like the south end of a cat goin' north."

"Okay." I turned to Sam. "Do you know what problem your wife's talking about?" Sam stared at the floor. Now I had two oysters to deal with. I took a deep breath and exhaled slowly—go with the resistance.

"Mrs. Hoag, may I call you Clemmie?" She nodded. "I apologize for asking personal questions. You don't know me, and I don't blame you for not wanting to talk about your private business with a stranger."

Clemmie settled back in her chair, so I continued. "Things that go on behind closed doors are nobody's business but your own. So, rather than that, would it be all right if we just spent some time getting to know each other?"

She nodded. Sam let out a deep sigh. One way to get insight

about a couple's dynamics is to ask the couple to tell the story of how they met. Sometimes, retelling their story evokes fond memories; sometimes not, but it was worth a shot.

"You all have been married for 40 years. How did you meet?"

Sam leaned toward me. "I was comin' back up the river in my boat, fixin' to sell my oysters at the dock. Well, I see Clemmie standin' in the river up to her tits in 40-degree water, diggin' for clams. Right then, I knew—that's the girl for me."

Clemmie looked sideways at Sam. A smile flitted at the corner of her mouth.

"What happened next?"

"Old coot nearly ran me down," Clemmie said.

"Then what?"

"I took a big sack of oysters to her house," Sam said.

"Then what?"

Clemmie took up the story. "My father opened the door, grabbed the bag of oysters, and threw Sam off the porch." She was smirking.

"Son of a bitch hated my guts."

"How come he didn't like you?"

"He said no goddamned Hoag was comin' near his daughter, and, if I knew what was good for me, I'd get the hell off his property and go back to the pigsty with the rest of the 'Hogs.'"

Clemmie chimed in. "Sam's grandfather shot my daddy's father over a piece of land they both wanted, so the Hoags and Painters never got along after that."

"So how did you two get together?"

"The next time I seen Sam, I was clammin' on the flats, so here comes Sam in his boat, and he starts yellin' at me, then he pulls out his gun, and I'm thinkin' he's crazy 'cuz he aims it at me and fires. I hear a splash and see a big ole 'gator thrashin' in the reeds. So, then I wade out to the boat, and he grabs me up. After that, my daddy couldn't say anythin' bad about Sam 'cause he saved my life." It looked like she wasn't even conscious that, at that point, she was patting Sam on the arm.

Sam was blushing. Beneath the hangdog ruin of the man, I saw the once-dashing Romeo.

"Clemmie, how old were you when this happened?"

"She was sixteen."

"Do you all have any children?"

"Two..." Clemmie dropped her head and paused. "We had two."

"Any grandchildren?"

"Two," she said.

"What're their names?"

"Cynthia and Billy Two. My daughter, Maria, named him after her brother."

Sam chimed in. "I'll tell you, that boy is smart—smarter'n me."

It was one of the few times I saw Sam smile. When I looked back at Clemmie, I saw a tear drop onto the alligator purse on her lap. She opened it, took out a hankie, and wiped her eyes.

Sam leaned forward. "She's thinkin' about Billy."

Clemmie nodded and blew her nose, then reached into her purse again, pulled out a photo, and handed it to me. It showed a handsome young man wearing a Marine Corps uniform.

"So handsome," I said to Clemmie.

"He's dead." Her voice and face were as flat as the photo.

"Sonsabitches killed my boy." Sam's whole body tensed. Clemmie stopped patting his arm and, instead, tightened her grip as if to keep him from bolting out of his chair.

"I'm so sorry. Who thinks they'll ever have to bury their child?" I paused. "How old was he?"

Clemmie answered. "Thirty-two."

Sam's voice was angry and tight. He stood up, leaned forward, and slapped the desk hard with his palms. "Sonsabitches put him in jail. Never did nothin' 'cept pick up a dead iggle. *Put him in a jail*! Didja know it's a federal offense to pick up a dead iggle? *Feder-al oh-fence*." Sam stood. His face was purple.

I was struggling to figure out what an iggle was. "Iggle?"

Flapping his arms, Sam took a step toward my desk. "A *iggle*..."

I was incredulous. "Billy went to jail for picking up a dead *eagle*?"

"*Goddamned right!*" Sam was shouting. Clemmie leaned forward and tugged on Sam's shirt. He turned and stomped over to the window.

She leaned toward me. "Last year, Billy was out huntin' in the Glades and found a dead eagle. So, he put it in his truck and figured he'd take it over to his friend, Carl Bullis, 'cause Carl's a Seminole and they use the feathers for a bunch of things. When Billy got back to town, he stopped at the 7-Eleven for gas. Sheila Bullis, Carl's sister, was workin' the cash register, and so Billy tells her he's got an eagle for Carl. Well, one of the park rangers who was in the store hears him and goes out and sees the dead eagle in Billy's truck and arrests him. Put him in handcuffs and everything right there."

"Why did he arrest him? Billy didn't kill it."

Sam stormed back over to my desk and, pronouncing each word slowly, said, "*It's a fed-er-al offense to possess a iggle even if you didn't kill it!*"

I asked, "There's a law about picking up dead eagles?"

Sam snorted and stomped back over to the window. He stood staring at the slate gray sky. Wind was starting to whip the palm tree fronds into a frenzy. I lost track of the session for a second to wonder if I'd make it home before the storm broke loose. Part of me also recognized it was the storm that was brewing in the office I wanted to escape.

Clemmie said, "Can't have an eagle 'less ya got a permit from the gov'mint." Her comment brought me back to the session. Sam stood across the room, staring out the glass door. His arms were folded and, even from the back, I could see his shoulders were tensed. The wind picked up. A huge, dead palm frond flew across the patio.

"But it was dead," I said, struggling to understand how possessing a dead bird could be illegal.

"Don't matter," Clemmie said. "Gotta have permit, else you can go to jail and get a fine."

Sam shouted from across the room, "Sentenced my boy to six months in prison and slapped him with a $10,000 fine for a damn dead bird. F--kin' gov'mint. They knew he couldn't pay the fine. Sent him up there on a Thursday. We didn't even get to see him before he went."

Clemmie picked up the story. "Got a visit from the sheriff on the following Monday. Came to tell us Billy was dead."

"What?" I was having a hard time taking in what they were telling me.

Clemmie said, "As soon as the sheriff drove up to the house, I knew right then. He steps up on the porch, takes off his hat, sez to me, 'Ma'am, I'm sorry to tell you, but your son, Billy Hoag, died yesterday.'"

"Oh, Clemmie," I said, "what happened?"

"He choked to death on a ham sandwich." Her voice broke. She covered her mouth with her wadded-up hankie.

Her story was surreal. *Your son finds a dead bird, goes to prison, and chokes to death on a ham sandwich? What the hell can I say to that?*

"They fined him. It seems harsh to send him to jail. Was it his first offense?"

Clemmie looked at Sam. "You tell her."

Sam stomped across the room, stopped at my desk, and then threw himself into his chair.

"Sam and Billy already done time," she said. "When they shut down the oyster beds, we didn't have any way to make money. So..."

Sam sat up. He pushed his hat back and fixed me eye to eye. "Five years ago, me and Billy was haulin' marijuana and got caught. I swear to God, I didn't want to, but a man's gotta feed his family...right?"

I nodded, because I agreed with him. If my family was in danger of starving, I'd do whatever to keep them alive. I glanced outside. The ibis flock sailed off, looking like so many pieces of paper scattered by the wind. I had to consciously refocus on what Sam was saying.

"So, we was unloadin' a delivery back in the mangroves and damn if the Feds didn't light us up and throw us in jail. I did eighteen months, and Billy did the same. But we didn't snitch on anybody else, so the Feds and the sonsabitches were just waitin' for any excuse to haul us in again."

Clemmie sat bolt upright. "I told him and told him—"

Sam whipped around and shouted, "*Shut up!*"

Clemmie flinched and pulled herself into herself, like a frightened turtle.

Sam stood and stormed out of the room. Clemmie looked up at me as if to say, "See what I'm living with?" I thought it was okay for Sam to go outside; give him a chance to calm down. I'd go get him back in a few minutes. In the meantime, I could talk to Clemmie alone.

"Has he always been like that?" I asked.

"Not before Billy died. He was a good provider, didn't hit me or the kids, liked to take a drink now and then, but he's gone mean since Billy. I told him if he didn't do somethin', I was gonna move up to Apalachicola with Maria and the kids."

The death of a child is cataclysmic. Grief and rage were tearing Sam and Clemmie apart. And lurking at the edge of grief were the twin devils, homicide and suicide. I still thought Sam had the potential to go off the deep end, maybe take revenge on the ranger or the judge or, if he got drunk enough, decide to put a bullet in his own head. At that thought, the hair on my body stood up, and my stomach knotted. I was afraid to ask the next question.

"Clemmie, where does Sam keep his guns?" She pressed her lips tightly together. "Are you afraid he's going to kill himself? Is that why you made him come here?"

She nodded. "He sits in the truck and drinks till he passes out. I try to get him to come inside." She was crying. "He keeps Billy's pistol on the seat beside him. Last week, I came out to check on him, and he had the pistol in his hand, and he was cryin', and I begged him to come in but..."

Something bad was about to happen. My stomach felt like I was falling down an elevator shaft. Adrenaline shot through my system.

"How did you and Sam get to the clinic today?"

Clemmie almost whispered, "In the truck."

My mind began to run at warp speed. *Press the alarm button under my desk and alert security, or go look for him myself?* Hesitating for a second, I thought, *If I send security to find Sam, I'm afraid he'll see them as "gov'mint." And, if he's armed, it's a crapshoot he'll decide to make a stand in the parking lot. I don't want to take that chance.* It didn't occur to me then that he might decide to shoot me.

"Clemmie. Wait here, I'll be back in a second." I ran down the hall.

Maybe he was in the waiting room. No Sam. I turned to Peg at the reception window. "Did you see Sam Hoag go by?"

"No."

I pushed open the door to the outside. The sky was turning blue-black. The wind was picking up. The palm trees were waving frantically. There were about six pickup trucks in the parking lot. Way off at the back corner, parked under a live oak, I saw someone sitting in a beat-up red Ford. Hurrying across the blacktop, toward the truck, I prayed. *God, please help.*

Sam was sitting in his truck, drinking a long-neck beer.

"Hey, Sam." No matter that he was a beer-drinking oysterman who'd done a stint in prison, I believed that, at heart, Sam was still a southern gentleman. He glanced out his window. I was out of breath and dripping with sweat.

"Got another one of those?" I pointed to the beer.

Totally inappropriate to ask an alcoholic client for a beer, but, at that point, I hoped the shock of his therapist asking for a beer would disrupt whatever else he might have been planning. He rolled down his window and passed me a beer. I lifted it in a "here's to you" gesture and pretended to take a slug.

"Good," I said and wiped the bottle across my face. I stood leaning against the fender. In the distance, I saw Peg and Clemmie looking at us across the parking lot. I waved at them to go back and hoped to God they'd stay away. The sky was the color of a bruise. Thunder rumbled in the distance.

Sam drained his bottle and belched. I held my breath for a second. "You ready to go back in?"

He sat staring out the windshield. Neither of us moved. A minute stretched out to forever. Since I'd walked across the parking lot, I'd never stopped praying, *God, please help*, because I knew for sure Sam had a gun. I wavered between trying to slide out of sight and trying to think of something that might buy me some time. Fat drops of rain spattered on the ground.

"Sam, what's Billy Two gonna feel like when he finds out his granddad killed himself?"

Sam didn't move for a long time. Then he leaned down below the window. My heart almost exploded. When he reappeared, I felt the blood drain from my head.

He opened the truck door and stepped out. Just before he closed it, I saw the butt of a revolver sticking out from under the seat. We walked back toward the clinic.

Just as we made it to the foyer, the rain came. The sound of it hitting the tin roof of the clinic was deafening. Clemmie was waiting inside with Peg, who gave me the "are you out of your mind?" look.

"Peg, we're fine. Clemmie, Sam, let's go back to my office."

Sam sat in the armchair. Clemmie pulled her chair closer to Sam's.

"Sam, you know why Clemmie made you come here, right?"

"Thinks I'm gonna kill myself."

"Yep. That's what she's afraid of. Sam, I don't think anybody would blame you for feeling like that. You got screwed by the government, your boy died because of a stupid law, your business is in the tank...I don't know how you stood it. But the thing is... what is Clemmie gonna tell Billy Two if you kill yourself? What's that little boy gonna tell his friends when they find out his grandpa killed himself? Billy Two already lost his uncle. How's he going to grow up without his grandpop?"

I had few scruples about what I'd say to someone who was seriously contemplating suicide. When it comes to suicide, it's all about keeping the person alive until hope returns. Over the years, I've found that often parents and grandparents will do something for their kids that they would never be willing to do for themselves. So, for the time being, if Sam would stay alive to spare his grandson from suffering and humiliation, that was the deal I'd make.

I pulled out the Contract for Safety that Sam had signed. "Can I share this with Clemmie?"

Sam nodded.

I told Clemmie, "This is an agreement that Sam won't kill himself. But he'll call 911 or the Suicide Prevention hotline if he starts to think about killing himself...or anybody else." I turned to Sam. "Sam, will you be willing to give Clemmie your guns to hold?"

He balked. "I said I wouldn't kill myself."

"I know, and I believe you, but—"

Clemmie interrupted. "You give me them guns or you ain't comin' home. I'll give 'em to Cliff to hold, and you can have 'em back later."

Sam shrugged. He looked too tired to argue anymore. "Okay, okay."

"Sam, if there's some medicine that might help you feel better, would you be willing to see our psychiatrist here?"

He frowned. Clemmie looked at me. "He'll see him."

"Sam? Can I have Clemmie make the appointments for follow-up?"

He nodded again.

"Clemmie," I said, "you are a very strong person—"

Sam interrupted. "You can say that again."

"And I want you to know I'm here for you as well as Sam. I'd like a chance to talk to you next time about how you're feeling."

Clemmie nodded once. When she stood up, I put my hand lightly on her arm.

"You can make the next appointments with Peg at the front desk."

Clemmie looked at Sam. "Come on, old man." She dropped her hankie into her alligator purse and snapped it shut.

Sam heaved himself out of the chair, hitched up his saggy shorts, and followed Clemmie, shuffling his way down the hall.

I breathed a huge sigh of relief. *Thank you, God*. It was 6:15 p.m. I tidied my desk, flipped off the light, and walked down the hall. It was pouring. The streets would be flooded. All of a sudden, I was so tired. I sat down in the empty lobby and stared out the window, wondering how it could happen that a man finds a dead bird, and that leads to his death.

The rest of the story

Sam kept his appointment with the psychiatrist, took medication for a little while, but got really pissed off when he found out the antidepressants he was taking were to blame for his lack of sexual arousal, so he quit taking them. Clemmie wasn't thrilled. She'd enjoyed a timeout from Sam "pesterin' me every darn night," but at least she and Sam were spending time fishing together. Sam didn't quit drinking but eased back on it.

At our last appointment, Clemmie reported they were planning a trip to Apalachicola to see the grandchildren. I stood up and came around the desk to say goodbye to them. Sam stuck out his hand, looked me in the eye, and said, "This wasn't so bad." I was touched. That was high praise indeed from a crusty oysterman.

10

RIP-OFF

You never know what the day will bring. Tuesday morning brought me David Cooper. He had been arrested for assault on a neighbor and was referred for counseling by the court. I met him in the waiting room. Blond hair, blue eyed, wearing a short-sleeved shirt with a button-down collar, he looked like a Bible salesman.

I introduced myself, and David followed me down the hall to my office. He sat down across from my desk, leaned forward, and said quietly, "You know, I could rip your face off."

Well, that was a showstopper. In all my years as a clinician, I'd been called names, threatened once or twice, but never so graphically. I debated. Should I just leave, or stay and see where this was going? Back in the day, one of my professors gave me some advice, which I've always followed: never sit between a client and the door, because there's something subliminally reassuring when a client sees they can easily leave the room. If things get too overwhelming, they don't feel trapped. And the added bonus is, if a client becomes threatening, you can also leave the room without having to pass by the client.

My desk was set up just to the right of the door; two steps and I was out of there. Aside from his bizarre remark, David's body language was relaxed. He sat calmly, looking at me. Because my curiosity overrode good sense, I decided to stay. I took a deep breath.

"And you would do that because…?"

He laughed. "I just wanted to see what you'd do."

I mentally called him a bunch of names but managed to sit and just nod.

He could laugh about testing me with that opening remark, but it was so dark and creepy, I didn't need to be Dr. Phil to know there was something very wrong with this guy—think Norman Bates. I had a cold knot in my stomach.

"So, you've been referred by the court?" I said.

He nodded once. His lack of affect was almost reptilian.

"Where else have you been seen?" I figured this cool customer probably had a long history of screwing around with therapeutic referrals, so asking where else he had been seen assumed he was experienced with courts and clinics, and maybe if he rattled off other locations, I'd get a better picture of his criminal and psychiatric history.

"I saw the prison shrink once a month."

His blink rate was very slow. The knot in my stomach tightened. The same professor who told me never to sit between a client and the door gave me another great piece of advice: always trust your gut. The knot in my stomach was affirmation that the guy sitting across from me wasn't just a shy, young man who'd somehow gotten a little lost. I was having a conversation with a convicted felon who'd qualified to see a forensic psychiatrist on a regular basis.

"Where was that?" I asked.

"YOI."

"Which was…?"

"Youthful Offender Institute."

"How old were you when you went in?"

"Fourteen."

Maybe it was his cold-blooded demeanor, coupled with the

slow eye blink, that evoked in me the image of a boa constrictor lying motionless on a tree branch, waiting for prey to pass by. "How long were you there?"

"Seven years." His affect and voice were totally flat.

"That seems like a long time for someone so young. How would you feel about telling me why you were in YOI?" Asking how he'd feel about telling me left David the option of not disclosing the specific traumatic event.

He ignored the question and seemed to have no reticence about telling me straight out what he'd done to garner such a long juvenile sentence.

"I killed my mother." He had a slight smile on his face, like he was enjoying his fantasy that his confession would freak me out.

I am rarely at a loss for words. However, this time was an exception. At that point, I might have finessed the next few questions, summed up my recommendations, and referred him to our shrink. But I didn't do that. They say curiosity killed the cat, but, since I wasn't a cat, I ventured further into the darkness.

Maybe David had had a reason for killing his mother. A bizarre concept for some, but each of us has our breaking point, and I wondered if David, as a young teen, may have suffered some outrageous kinds of punishment, or humiliation, or sexual abuse at the hands of his mother. People who haven't ever had evil touch their lives might be offended by my thinking that, but, over the years, I've learned there is no limit to what one human being will do to another.

"What happened?"

"I hit her with an ax."

I started to feel nauseous. "Then what?" I asked.

"Then nothing. I got busted."

So, there I sat, an older woman, wearing glasses, a little pudgy, a little gray—in short, the motherly type. I wasn't the therapist for David. His demeanor, coupled with the feeling in my gut, told me that whatever was going on with him was way beyond my pay grade; besides, the issues of transference and countertransference would be way too sticky for me. I decided to complete the interview then refer him to Bob Sutton, one of our clinic psychiatrists, for a full evaluation.

"David, thank you for being forthcoming. I'm going to refer you for an evaluation with our psychiatrist here, Dr. Sutton. He's a good guy. I know you've already had extensive counseling, but maybe he can help you work out some of the issues with the court."

"Okay."

I pushed back from my desk and stood up. "Let's go up front so we can make the appointment for Dr. Sutton."

David remained in his seat. I saw a defiant four-year-old smirking, challenging me with an unsaid "make me."

I looked at him and smiled. "Come on, it's almost lunchtime." I reached over, flipped off the light, and walked out of the room. I heard him push back his chair. The entire time he was following me up the hall, my heart was in my throat. He stopped behind me at the desk, and I handed him off to Peg so she could make an appointment for him with Bob.

The rest of the story

I don't scare easily. I'm sure there were a hundred other things someone else might have done that might have been more therapeutic for David, but he touched some fear in me that lingered. For several months afterward, when I had evening hours, I made sure someone always walked me to my car.

In my opinion, the justice system today is skewed. The concept of good and evil no longer prevails. The prevailing belief is that rehabilitation is the answer. People think there's some kind of magic in therapy and, given the right mix of counseling and/or meds, everyone can be rehabilitated. There are many who have run afoul of the law and, once they've served their sentence, come out changed for the better. But they don't generally meet the criteria for sociopath or psychopath.

If the person doesn't want to change, or has significant psychopathic tendencies, then, barring divine intervention, chances of rehabilitation are slim.

Watch the nightly news following the trial and conviction of a serial killer or someone who's been found guilty of a heinous murder. After the verdict, the poor family always looks bewildered, and, invariably, they want to ask just one question of the murderer. In poignant, tear-filled voices, they all ask the same thing: Why?

Why? If the killer was willing to answer honestly, they'd say one of three things: I felt like it, I enjoyed it, or because I could. There are some kinds of behaviors that no amount of therapy or meds will ever change.

I never did hear the outcome of David's case. I followed up with Bob, the psychiatrist, but, due to some legal issues, the case dragged on for a long time, and other folks came for treatment in that time, and I lost track of David. I imagine he's still living in the community. I've often said to Alex that, if people ever knew who walks among us freely, they'd never leave their homes.

11

GOD HELP US

Friday, 5:30 a.m.

"This just in: A massive explosion has leveled an abortion clinic in Miami. Four confirmed dead, many injured."

I glanced at the TV. Emergency vehicles, red and blue strobe lights flashing, were parked helter-skelter around a rubble-strewn site.

"More at six."

Monday morning, 7:45 a.m.

Driving to work, the news was all about the bombing.

"The FBI reports that nineteen-year-old Harold Clayton is being sought in the bombing of the abortion clinic in Miami. He was arrested last year for an alleged attempt to assassinate a doctor who ran an abortion clinic in Colorado; however, charges were dropped. Anyone knowing his whereabouts is asked to call their local police or FBI agency."

I pulled into my spot at the Palmetto Behavioral Health Clinic. Once inside the lobby, the AC was so cold, my glasses fogged up. I said hi to Peg, the receptionist, then ambled down the hall to my office. As soon as I opened the door, I spotted the note propped on my desk: Come see me ASAP—ML.

I walked down the hall to my supervisor, Martha Legget.

"Hey," she said, "how was your weekend?"

"Good."

"You heard about the bombing at the abortion clinic?"

"Yes."

"Harold Clayton's mother is in our crisis unit."

"Harold Clayton—the bomber guy? His mother is in the crisis unit?" I sounded stupid, but the fact that the mother of the man wanted for bombing a clinic in Miami was in our psychiatric crisis unit was, well, mind-blowing.

"Her husband brought her in last night. Phil did the intake. I'd like you to do an assessment, and then we'll figure out what's going on."

"Okay. Let me check my messages and talk to Peg about my schedule."

"I'll see whoever you have this morning, or we'll reschedule them. I want you to see Mary Clayton as soon as you can."

"Is Phil in yet? I'd like to talk to him before I see her."

"I think I saw his Corvette in the parking lot."

I hurried down the hall to Phil's office. The sign on his door said "Phillip Pomeroy, M.D. Medical Director." I knocked.

"Yo, come in."

Phil's office had the same basic, public mental health clinic décor we all had: gray metal desk, two office chairs facing said desk, and a bookcase flanking the window. On the wall beside his desk, he had a wild Miro print titled *The Singing Fish*.

Phil, wearing khakis and Top-Siders, no socks, feet up on his desk, was dictating a progress note. I stood there waiting for him to finish. He pushed his black-rimmed glasses up on his bald head and swung his feet off the desk.

"So—Mary Clayton, right? Okay, so you know her son bombed the clinic in Miami, right?"

"Well, it sounds like he's the guy."

"Yeah, trust me. He's the guy. The father said he was afraid of something like this."

I sat down in the chair across from the desk. "What's the story?"

"The husband brought the mother in—poor guy. He didn't want to talk about himself, just hyper-focused on the wife; she was almost catatonic. Couldn't or wouldn't talk, glassy stare...no affect. I figured she'd taken something, but husband says not. He told me she was seeing a guy for anxiety and depression before they moved here, and she'd been hospitalized once about four years ago for depression." He ran his hand over his head. "Given the situation, I thought it wouldn't hurt to give her a look-see— might help keep the news vultures from hounding her, at least for a little while."

"Have you seen her yet this morning?"

"No, I just got here and finished dictating the admission note. The dad said Harold has always been a little 'different.'" Lost in thought, he fiddled with a paper clip and shook his head. "Sad."

"Martha wants me to see her. D'you want to come along, or d'you want me to see you after I see her?"

"Yeah, you go see her and come back and tell me what you think."

I took the back entrance from the clinic, crossed a courtyard, and buzzed the crisis unit buzzer. Jose Camacho, the unit aide, opened the door. His Jack o' lantern smile was infectious.

"Hey, Jose. How're you doing?"

"Pretty good. You know who we got in last night?"

"Mary Clayton. That's who I'm here to see."

"Poor lady," he said. I followed him down the hall. He stopped at door number one and unlocked it.

"Ms. Clayton," he said, "Ms. Bugaeff, the social worker, is here to see you."

Mary Clayton sat slumped on the edge of her bed. Her hair was a faded blond. Her skin was ashen. She lifted her head in slow motion, like one of the animatronic figures they have at Disney World. Her pale blue eyes stared through me.

"Thanks, Jose. I'll knock when I'm ready to leave." I stood in the doorway for a second. "Mary," I said quietly, "my name is Pinny Bugaeff. I'm a social worker."

Mary was somewhere far away and, given what she was facing, I wasn't sure I wanted to bring her back. I went over and sat down next to her bed.

"Mary." I reached over and took her hand. It was cold. "Mary, I've heard what happened. I'm so sorry."

She began to rock. I put my other hand gently on her arm to get her attention.

"Mary? Do you know where you are?"

"Hospital?" she whispered.

"Do you know which hospital?"

"Umm...mental hospital."

"Do you know what day it is?"

She thought for a minute. "Monday?"

"Right. It's Monday, and you're in the Palmetto Behavioral Health Clinic."

She looked down and nodded.

"Your husband was worried about you and brought you here. Do you know why?"

"Harold." She buried her face in her hands. "He killed all those people." A wrenching howl of pain bounced off the walls. I prayed I'd find a way to help her live through this.

After a long while, her sobs subsided. She drew a shaky, deep breath and swiped her nose on the sleeve of her faded-green johnny gown. I reached over to the bedside table, grabbed a handful of tissues, and handed them to her. She took them without looking at me. She wiped her eyes and blew her nose. Her hair hung in limp strands around her face.

"Where were you when you heard?" I asked.

"Home."

"Where's home?"

Slumped in despair, there was another long pause.

"Garden Cove. We just moved here."

"Where did you move from?"

"Minnesota."

"What made you decide to come to Florida?"

"My husband wanted to retire."

Her voice was devoid of intonation. At that point, all I was trying to do was establish a connection, to get her back into the present moment by asking simple, concrete questions.

"Did you work when you lived in Minnesota?"

"No…I volunteered…at church." She began slowly folding the hem of her gown into accordion pleats.

"Have you heard from anyone from your church yet?"

"Jim said Father Paul called. What must they think of me?" she whispered. "Harold—he killed all those people. I don't know what happened." Still not making eye contact, she asked, "Do you know if it was really him?"

"Once we finish here, I'll try and find out anything more that I can. I know you want to know what's going on."

She nodded slowly and smoothed the folds in the hem of her gown then, once again, began refolding it into pleats.

"Mary, can I ask you a few questions about Harold?"

She stopped the ritual folding and, as if trying to hold herself together, wrapped her arms around herself.

"What was Harold like as a child?" Still glassy-eyed, she took a long time before she spoke, almost a whisper.

"He was a good baby—hardly ever cried. All my friends complained, because their babies cried all the time, but Harold—he hardly cried at all."

I thought about what the neighbors always say when the boy

next door kills his mother with a hatchet: "He was such a nice, quiet boy."

"What was he like in school?"

"Oh, he did real well—kinda shy—but the Sisters loved him. They say he killed all those people at the abortion clinic." She burst into tears again. "Have they found him yet?"

"Not that I know of. I was listening to the radio on the way in."

"He did it," she mumbled. "I'm afraid he's going to do it again."

"What makes you think that?"

"He hated abortion, and I think the people he was with are…" She went silent and sat staring at the floor.

"Are what?"

Did she know there was going to be another bombing? If so, I might be getting into deep water. Although I was operating under strict regulations of confidentiality, this was another case, like Sam's, where the Tarasoff law might come into play. Was I getting into Duty-to-Warn territory? Granted, Mary was just speculating about a crime her son had committed, but, given his recent actions, I wanted to get his mother's perception about the likelihood of Harold continuing his killing spree.

It's not unusual that adults who kill often have a history of cruelty to pets or small animals, and, if they have that kind of history, that tends to figure in their adult potential for violence. I was trying to figure out if Harold was a zealot, psychopath, mentally ill, or maybe all three.

"Tell me more about Harold. Did he have pets?"

"Well, he was very quiet, like I said, hardly ever cried." Her voice was flat. "He was allergic to dogs and cats, so no pets. He spent hours in his room building things with Lego. He was an altar boy. Father Robert told me he might have the makings of a priest." Her voice was still flat. She sounded like she was in a trance, which in a way she was, but listening to her kicked my thought process into high gear.

"Did Harold have friends?"

"Well, he mostly liked to stay home. The boys in the neighborhood were awfully rough. But he was friends with Lydia, the girl next door. They went to catechism together. Her mother told me she hoped Lydia would become a nun." Mary looked like she was still in shock, but a little color was coming back to her face, and she was making more eye contact with me.

"What was Harold like as a teenager?"

She thought for a minute. "Well, that's when we sort of noticed he was changing."

"Changing?"

"He got real interested in the pro-life group at church. He started to go to Mass every day. He told everybody God told him they were going to Hell if they had an abortion. He loved babies so much…" She drifted off. I waited. "He also didn't like to change his clothes. His father practically had to drag him into the bathroom to take a shower."

My internal conversation was amping up. Harold's earlier history—hardly cried, few friends, religiosity; teen years—loner, deepening religious fervor, zeal about a cause, deterioration in hygiene; taken individually, or even as a whole, those things could apply to a lot of teenagers who weren't mentally ill. Given that Harold had told his mother that God told him to do it…and now he'd bombed the clinic, I was wondering if Harold was just a zealot or if he was hearing command hallucinations, which may be a sign a teen is perhaps experiencing the onset of schizophrenia or is maybe taking drugs.

"Did you and your husband ever take Harold for counseling for mental health or maybe," I hesitated, "drug problems?" Mary's head snapped up.

"Harold never took drugs." She said it with the conviction of a mother who would swear she knew her son inside and out and was appalled I'd even asked. However, there are a lot of teens who do things that would cause their parents to have apoplexy if they were found out.

"Well, we talked about counseling for his...other problems, but Father Paul said he'd talk to him and make sure he stayed busy. And he said he'd say a Mass for him."

Mary was a rare bird, a guileless and gentle soul, unworldly—a good Catholic wife and mother. If the priest said he'd take care of her son and all Harold needed was to be kept busy, that was sufficient reassurance for her.

"Did you notice anything else unusual about Harold? Did he ever say anything that made you wonder why the heck he was saying that? Or maybe he had some ideas that struck you as a little odd or different than other kids his age?"

She sat there thinking then looked up at me. She pushed her straggly hair away from her face. Her pale blue eyes were red from crying. "One night, I was sitting in the kitchen, and he came in and said somebody was talking about him. So, I told him there wasn't anybody else here, and he got real mad and said, 'You have to tell them to stop saying things about me.' I guess I thought he was trying to play a trick on me, but I couldn't get him to calm down, and then he got really quiet and went up to his room." Mary bowed her head and resumed pleating her hem.

"Did he ask you any other time about maybe seeing or hearing something that wasn't there?"

"Once he was at K-Mart with his dad and asked him if he saw the black fox. Jim told me Harold got really angry when he told him there was no black fox loose in K-Mart."

"How old was he when he started asking about seeing the fox?"

"Hmm. Maybe fifteen?"

Now I had a report of both auditory and visual hallucinations. If mental illness was driving him, rather than zeal, that would be important information, both now and for later, when Harold might be facing charges. I continued to speculate. Mary reported that Harold was a loner, had intensified religiosity, and was in the grip of an obsession about abortion. He'd shown disregard for personal hygiene and was reporting what sounded like hallucinations.

A lot of people might write off those clues as applicable to a bad case of teenage angst, but the more I heard, the stronger the feeling I got that Harold might in fact be suffering from paranoid schizophrenia. Of course, I hadn't seen him, so no use jumping to conclusions, because everything at that point was just preliminary.

"When did you last see Harold?"

"We stopped in to see him in Tennessee, on the way to Florida."

"What was he doing there?"

"Well, he'd followed one of the church members down to help do some volunteer work."

"What kind of volunteer work?"

"There's a big Right to Life movement at this church, and Harold was going to be helping, so his dad and I stopped in to see him...to see if he was okay, because we couldn't get a hold of him on the phone."

She stopped talking, and her voice dropped to a whisper. "So, we went to his apartment, but it was all closed up. We called him from the car, but he didn't answer his phone, so Jim went up and knocked and knocked real loud on the door. We thought he might be in there, but we got scared, so we called the church where he was volunteering, and they said they hadn't seen him for a week."

"So, what did you do?"

"His dad finally found the landlord, and he let us into Harold's apartment." Mary started rocking again.

"Can you tell me what was going on?" I hated to push, but as long as Harold wasn't in custody, I was afraid there might be more lives at stake.

Mary, rocking slowly, stared at the floor, her voice so whispery, I had to bend my head to hear her.

"All his windows were covered in aluminum foil—the ceiling, the walls, everything..."

Comedians make fun of people who wear tinfoil hats, but, sadly, there is some truth in their jokes. I've seen more than a few people who felt their thoughts were being controlled or monitored and used tinfoil on their windows to try to block their thought waves from getting out or to block evil forces from coming in.

"The apartment was filthy." She covered her mouth with her hand and continued rocking. "Whoever thinks their boy is going to kill people? He was a good boy." She was silently sobbing. I didn't have the heart to remind her he'd once been arrested for attempted murder of the doctor in Colorado.

"Mary, do you have any relatives in Florida, besides your husband?" I figured either Harold would be captured and eventually tried, which would be a massive ordeal, or he'd be killed attempting to evade arrest. In either case, Mary was going to need support to survive the coming days.

"My sister lives in Orlando."

"Mary, when I go back to the clinic, I'm going to call Jim and set up a time so we can get together and talk about how you're going to all get through this. Is he coming in to see you today?"

"I don't know. He's so worried…I think he said he was talking to the FBI."

"Would you like a visit from a priest?"

"I don't know any from around here." She sounded like a tired little girl. My heart went out to her.

"I do. Father Jake is a friend of mine. Would you like me to see if he can come in for a visit?"

She nodded, then reached over, grabbed my hand, and looked me in the face. "Will they kill him?"

I couldn't give her an honest answer. The probability of Harold's capture ending in death was pretty high. I figured that, given his mental state and the severity of his crime, if he was cornered, there was a pretty good chance he wouldn't surrender quietly. He had a lot of the hallmarks of a guy who might choose martyrdom or suicide by cop. I didn't want to lie to Mary, and nor did I want to destroy what little hope she might have. I silently said the prayer I pray when I'm out of answers, *God, please help*. Sure enough, I heard His answer. *Pray with her*. At the time, I was aware of the irony that Harold may not have been the only one hearing God's voice.

"Mary, would you like us to say a prayer for Harold?"

She nodded slowly. We bowed our heads.

"God," I began, "Harold is your child. He is in danger and needs Your help. We pray that You will stand between him and all harm, and You will hold him in the palm of Your hand until he finds his way to peace and safety."

I don't as a rule pray out loud with my clients, but as a person of faith, if a client such as Mary lives a life of faith, I feel that offering to pray with that person is sometimes the best support I can offer. Mary let out an audible sigh. We sat side by side in silence for a long time.

"Mary? Have you slept since yesterday?"

She shook her head no.

"Can you lie down for a few minutes and rest? Dr. Pomeroy, our psychiatrist, will be coming in to see you. I'll call Father Jake and see when he can come in for a visit. After you rest, you can make some phone calls, and I'll see what I can arrange so that anyone else you want can come in to see you."

Mary sat like a rag doll, lost in despair.

The rest of the story

As things turned out, Harold was arrested a few days later, without incident. As part of pre-trial proceedings, he was seen by two forensic psychiatrists and diagnosed with paranoid schizophrenia. He was deemed unable to assist in his defense and was sent to the state hospital, confined to the forensic ward for the criminally insane.

I continued to see Mary and Jim through all the phases of Harold's arrest and confinement in the hospital. They were people of deep faith but, each time they returned from a visit with

Harold, they suffered the aftershocks of having seen their only son wandering the dayroom, lost and disheveled, still ranting against abortion. They struggled to understand how or why paranoid schizophrenia had been visited upon their only child, but eventually they came to accept that Harold was the victim of a severe brain disorder. However, that did little to assuage their feelings of grief for their son and for his victims.

A year to the day of the clinic bombing, Harold committed suicide. After the private funeral service ended, I was standing on the church steps. Mary came over. We embraced.

"He's safe now," she whispered.

12

KENNY THE FARTING ANGEL

Kenneth Harrington Baines III. Age 26. I saw his name on the intake sheet and imagined a preppy, Ivy League type. Figuring I'd be able to easily spot the scion of the Baines family, I went down the hall to the waiting room. There were three candidates to choose from: a blond wearing flip flops, who was sprawled on the couch; an old guy wearing a T-shirt that said Pull my Finger; and a young man wearing a Chemise Lacoste golf shirt. He was picking his nose. Could this be Kenneth Harrington Baines the Third?

"Mr. Baines?"

He bounced out of his chair.

"Yep. That's me! Call me Kenny." He stuck out his hand. The same hand that had recently been mining his nose. I gave it a quick shake. Once more, the mantra about not assuming anything was proven. I led the way down the hall, back to my office.

Kenny plopped down in the chair across from my desk. His feet barely touched the floor. I guessed he might be slow.

"Kenny, my name is Pinny." I smiled at him. "Have you ever been in counseling before?"

"Yep."

At that point, Kenneth Harrington Baines III leaned to one

side, lifted his left butt cheek off the chair, and let out a very loud fart. Then, with a beatific smile, settled back, ready to continue our conversation.

My first reactions—shock and surprise—almost made me laugh. Kenny showed no signs of embarrassment. I decided to ignore it—assume the poor guy was nervous, maybe experiencing some kind of digestive upset. But this breech of social mores was another clue Kenny might be slow.

Attempting to restart the interview, I asked, "Kenny, why have you been in counseling before?"

"'Cuz I can't get a girlfriend." He was so downcast, he reminded me of Eeyore.

I was pretty sure I knew why Kenny couldn't get a girlfriend, but, still, I really wanted to find out more about this sweet little guy.

"Did you have any luck getting a girlfriend after you had counseling?"

His face scrunched up. "Nope."

"Did you ever figure out why you've had such a hard time?"

"Yeah. Girls don't like me." His face scrunched up, and he looked like he was going to cry.

My heart went out to him. He might not be the tall, dark, handsome Ivy Leaguer his name implied, but surely there are tons of folks who aren't picture-book perfect who find partners.

"Do you live in your own place?"

"Yep, I got a condo. Me and Bill share."

"Who's Bill?"

"He's the guy my mom and dad pay to keep an eye on me. They think I'm too dumb to live on my own." He paused. "They are kinda right 'cuz, like paying bills...and stuff, that's hard to do."

"Okay. Have you asked Bill about the girlfriend thing?"

"Yeah, but he just says, 'Ya can't trust bitches.'" He blushed when he said bitches, so maybe there was some sort of social awareness going on with him.

"Hmm. Do you think he's right?"

"Well, some girls are nice, but some are a bit…uh, you know."

Sadly, there are very few young women who are seeking little guys who pick their nose and fart loudly in public. "What have you tried to do to see if you can meet a girl?" (This incident took place long before there was an Internet, so that wasn't an option.)

"Me and Bill go to happy hour."

"How's that turned out for you?"

"Bad for me—good for Bill." Kenny was looking sadder by the minute.

I wondered if his parents, who were footing the bill, knew that Bill, the mentor, was looking for bitches at happy hour with their son.

At this point, Kenny lifted up on his butt cheek and let another fart fly. It was time for me to confront the elephant fart in the room. "Kenny, did your mom or dad ever say anything to you about farting?"

He snickered. "Yeah, my mother says it's rude, and I shouldn't do it."

"But you do it anyway?"

"Yep. It feels good." He smiled an impish smile.

"Kenny. Do you ever not fart, even if you feel like it?"

"Like in church?"

I nodded. "Like in church."

"Well. My mother told me God doesn't like it if people fart in church. So, I don't."

I shifted my focus to the scene outside the sliding glass door. The palm trees stood like giants, their fronds waving in the breeze, as if beckoning me to come outside and play. At that moment, I was wishing I could.

"Kenny." I hoped God would forgive me for what I was about to say, but I figured it was in a very good cause and was going to be a blessing—maybe. "Kenny, your mom is right. God doesn't like farting in church, and you do the right thing and show respect by not doing it. Now, I'm going to tell you something else about farting. Most girls don't like farting. Like it's disrespectful to God, it's also disrespectful to girls."

He looked stricken. "But Bill said it was funny, and girls think it's funny, too." The dialogue I was having with myself inside my head was something like, *Farting...I'm talking about farting! I went to six years of college to talk about farting.* I was laughing inside but also seething. Thanks to his roommate, Kenny totally believed farting was the way to a woman's heart. I bit my tongue, hard. At that moment, I wanted to kill Bill.

"Kenny," I said, "I know a whole lot of women—young women, smart women, kind women, tall women, short women, pretty women—all kinds of women, and the truth is, neither God nor women like farting."

Brow furrowed, Kenny looked at me. "Girls don't like farting?" He was sincerely bemused. "But Bill said…"

"Kenny, maybe Bill was joking with you." It galled me to make an excuse for the rat, but better not to upset the applecart just yet. "Truthfully, most girls really don't like farting."

Kenny still looked a little skeptical.

"If you ask your mom again, do you think she'll tell you the truth?"

"Yep. My mom says it's a sin to lie."

"Kenny, would it be okay with you if I had a meeting with your mom and dad to see if we can figure out how we can help you?"

"Yep. My mother was the one who said I should go back to counseling."

"So, I'll call up your mom, and we can make an appointment to get together with her and your dad. You know that what you told me today is private between you and me, right? But, if you say so, we can all talk about this."

"Yep, that's what Dr. Block said, too."

"Who is Dr. Block?" I wondered if that was his former therapist.

"Dr. Block is my doctor, and he operates on the drain thing in my head when the water in my brain gets too much."

Water in his brain. The puzzle pieces were starting to come together. It was likely Kenny had been born with hydrocephaly—commonly called water on the brain. Usually a shunt is installed to drain excess fluid into the abdomen or vein in the neck. When it occurs at birth, it can cause the kind of impairments I was seeing in Kenny.

"When your mom and dad come in, can I tell them what we talked about?"

"Farting?"

"Well, farting and girlfriends and stuff."

"Yep."

Kenny bounced off his chair, then followed me down the hall back to the waiting room.

"I'll call your mom and set up an appointment."

"Yep."

Just as Kenny pushed through the glass doors to the outside, a silver Jaguar pulled up. Kenny got in, and the Jag sped out of the parking lot.

―――

THE FOLLOWING TUESDAY, I WENT OUT TO MEET MARCIA, MRS. Kenneth Harrington Baines II, and her husband, "call me Ken," in the waiting room. Both looked to be in their 70s, and they looked like old money. Marcia was wearing a Lily Pulitzer cotton shift, and Ken wore a Chemise Lacoste golf shirt. They confirmed that Kenny, their only child, had, indeed, been born with hydrocephalus.

"I married late, and we never thought we'd have a baby," Marcia said. "But there I was, 42 years old and pregnant. We were so blessed, we called him our angel baby." Marcia showed no sign of regret that her angel had been born with hydrocephalus. Kenny's dad sat quietly, staring at the floor.

After a short discussion about Kenny and his history, I asked what they thought about the way Bill was working out. They got quiet and exchanged a glance. Most Midwesterners, I've found, are loath to say anything negative about anybody.

Marcia sighed and turned to her husband. "You tell her."

"Bill's my sister's son."

"What's Bill's story?"

"Bill's been in trouble since he was a little kid. When he got out of jail, Mary begged us to help him…" Ken Sr. pursed his lips and glanced at his watch, as if this meeting was already lasting too long. Or maybe he was so uncomfortable, he just wanted it to be over.

I noted to myself that both Ken Sr. and I were wishing we were someplace else. What was going on beneath the surface that we were avoiding?

"So, how do you think he's working out?"

They glanced at each other.

"Not good," Marcia said. "We knew about Bill, but it's not so easy to find someone who wants to live with…um…you know… but we thought, since Bill is family, it might be all right." Ken slumped in his chair, head down.

"Have you talked to Kenny about his girlfriend issues?"

"Yep." Now Ken Sr. sounded like Eeyore Sr. "Kid wants a girlfriend…can't blame him…but…"

"But what?"

"How the heck is he going to get a girlfriend?" Ken leaned toward me. His face got red; his voice got tight and louder. "He can't drive. He can hardly read, farts all the time…" Ken sounded angry, but it felt like his anger was a thin veneer laid over a very deep wound. I felt the sadness of a father who believes his only son would never fly.

"I'm sorry, I just…" His eyes filled with tears; he couldn't speak.

"Marcia, Ken, let me summarize things. You've done everything you can think of to help support Kenny in having as independent a life as possible, including providing a condo, a car, and a mentor, but, despite all that, Kenny is depressed and frustrated. And his normal desire for a girlfriend or even meaningful companionship with people his own age isn't working."

Ken said, "Not just that, but we're getting much older and we don't know what's going to happen when we're gone." Okay, so now the truth emerged. We were entering the death zone.

"Have you made plans for Kenny for when that day comes?"

Ken's tone was terse. "We've got a trust set up, and our lawyer has papers that give him guardianship of Kenny."

"So far, you all have been Kenny's full-time social service agency, but now, as you said, he's at a stage where his needs as a young adult are getting more complex, and none of us are getting any younger. What do you all know about the Association for Retarded Citizens?" (ARC is a national organization that advocates and provides resources for retarded citizens. I'm aware retarded is no longer a politically correct term, but it was originally what the R stood for in ARC.)

Ken looked at me with a jaundiced eye. "We know about ARC, but we don't want to take money from others that need it more than us."

I saw Marcia shoot a sidelong glance at her husband. Ken's face turned red.

"Is your reticence about using them more than the money thing?"

"Goddamned right it's more than money!" Ken stood up, turned, and marched out the door.

Marcia said, "He's never gotten over it."

"What's 'it'?"

"His only child is...retarded. Ken loves Kenny, in his own way, but he never got over..." She swallowed, and tears ran down her cheeks. "He never wanted to talk about it. That's why he always just pays for us to try and fix it."

This wasn't just Social Work 101. This wasn't just Kenny needing outside provider services, it was also about the shame and grief of a father who couldn't accept his son. But, as long as his parents could afford to keep him insulated from the world, Kenny's prospects of finding a girl or a job or a social life were slim to none.

"Marcia, has anyone ever suggested a parents' group for you or Ken?"

"Dr. Block did, and Ken hit the roof."

"What else have you tried to do to get social services for Kenny?"

"Back in Cincinnati, I signed him up for a special job-training program, but Ken was furious."

"Why?"

"He went to drop Kenny off, and, when he saw what the other guys in the program looked like, he turned around and brought Kenny back home because he didn't want his son to be with..." she whispered, "what he called freaks."

I felt for Ken Senior. Both times he'd seen his son among peers, he literally couldn't face it. But a father who really didn't love his son would have simply been indifferent. Ken was far from indifferent. His inability to talk about Kenny's intellectual challenges brought him to tears.

"Has Ken ever talked about Kenny's disabilities?"

She shook her head.

"What happens when you try to talk to him about it?"

"You saw."

It was time to go see if I could find Ken and bring him back to the session. He was sitting in the empty waiting room, leafing through a magazine.

"Ken, I'm sorry this is such a rough session. Would you come back to my office so we can wrap things up?"

He tossed the magazine on a table and followed me back to my office.

"Ken, I want to say, first of all, that I think you and Marcia have gone above and beyond for Kenny, but, despite your best efforts, he isn't really finding his way. And it seems a shame the very things you've been doing aren't getting Kenny into any kind of social situations, other than happy hours with Bill, who apparently has convinced Kenny that farting is the way to impress girls and that most girls are bitches."

"I knew it was a mistake to hire that SOB," Ken said. He turned to Marcia. "When we get home, I'm going over there to throw him out."

"Ken, Marcia, can I make a suggestion? As much as I sympathize with you all and the Bill situation, as far as I can tell, there's no crisis imminent. It's not an emergency; it's a lousy situation that needs to be fixed. Do you think it needs to be fixed immediately, or could you maybe buy yourselves some time to work out a solution for the Bill situation?"

Ken sat bolt upright. "Not one more damn minute for that SOB."

"Ken." Marcia verbally put her foot down. "We need to talk. Bill has had his chance, but let's not be too hasty before we've got our ducks in a row."

He growled but seemed to acquiesce by nodding agreement with Marcia.

I leaned toward them. "Ken, Marcia, would you be willing to come back in two weeks and, during that time, come up with a plan you think might work so that Kenny can have a social life, and you can get some peace of mind about plans for him?"

They nodded. We made a follow-up appointment, and they left.

The rest of the story

Two weeks later, I met with Ken Sr. and Marcia. After the preliminaries, I asked them to tell me what they'd thought about with regard to the Kenny situation.

Marcia spoke first. "We're going back to Cincinnati. Season here is almost over."

I hesitated. Did that mean they were just walking, or rather flying, away from the problem?

Marcia went on. "And we're taking Kenny back with us."

They must have seen the confusion on my face, because Ken interceded.

"What you said last week about Bill...well...we knew something like that was going on, but the whole situation is a rat's nest. So, we're taking Kenny back to Cincinnati, and we're going to tell Linda, my sister, that Kenny needs some additional follow-up and tests with his neurologist, and we're closing the condo."

"Last time we were here," Marcia said, "when we left, Ken was so angry, he said he was never coming back."

Nodding, I waited for her to continue, or for Ken to give me a piece of his mind for stirring up such painful issues. After a long silence, I said, "Yet here you both are."

Ken sighed deeply. "I'm just tired of trying..." He could barely speak. "...trying to make Kenny...into..." He swallowed back tears and turned to Marcia.

"He means he's never been willing to accept that Kenny is... who he is."

"I think a lot of dads might feel like that." I turned to Marcia. "Imagine that, all your life, you've dreamed of going to Italy, a sun-drenched country filled with wine and romance. When you finally board the plane for your once-in-a-lifetime trip, just before you land, they announce that, in fact, you're not getting your dream trip to Italy, but they've substituted a hike though the snowcapped Alps in Switzerland." I saw Ken out the corner of my eye, nodding almost imperceptibly.

"I'm never getting the trip to Italy." Ken's tone of voice verged between resignation and acceptance.

"And...so?" I looked at Marcia.

"And so, we're going to take Kenny back to Cincinnati and see if we can find someplace where he can make friends and get sheltered job training. Dr. Block has bugged us for years about going to the Deborah Center; it's got programs for people like Kenny. He can stay with us until we find some sort of services that he can still get...even when we're gone. Maybe a group home."

"Ken, how do you feel about taking this new path? Social Services...programs?"

He smiled ruefully and looked at me over the top of his glasses. "I'm getting too old to climb the Alps alone."

A month later, I got a call. It was Marcia. "We just want to thank you for seeing us. Kenny's started at a daytime job program in a sheltered workshop." Her voice broke. "Ken drives him there every morning."

13

GOTTA BUY A RAT

I was sitting at my desk in my office, waiting for my next client, Zulema Perez. I'd been seeing her on an outpatient basis for the past four months, trying to get her to agree to go into a residential program at the Oaks, a shelter for pregnant women. But, every time Zulema was about to come in, she'd disappear, and, when she came back, she always told the same story.

"Leo and me are getting married, and he's takin' me to Mexico, so I don't need couns'lin' no more."

I seriously doubted her story, since her scumbag boyfriend, Leo, had her turning tricks to pay for their drugs. Then she'd get arrested for soliciting, possession, or drunk and disorderly, tell the judge she was in counseling, and it would start all over. As much as she frustrated me, I had a soft spot for Zee.

"Mizz B...?" Zulema was standing in the doorway.

Her huge, brown eyes were almost covered by too-long, black bangs. Aged eighteen, she looked forty and was eight-and-a-half months pregnant. She smelled like cigarettes and hangover.

"Hi, Zee." The first day she'd come in, I'd called her Zulema.

"Miss, you can call me Zee."

"Just Zee?"

"Yeah, 'cause my first name starts with Z, and my last name ends with Z." She smiled and made a little joke. "It's easy."

She waddled over to the small wing chair across from my desk and plopped herself down, knees akimbo. I couldn't help but stare at her left leg which displayed a tattoo of a snake coiled around her calf, the head of which was hidden under Zee's skirt. There were dark circles under her eyes.

"You look tired," I said.

"Oh, my God," she replied. Tears welled in her eyes and ran down her cheeks. "You don't know. I was up all night looking for Leo's Sissy. I can't find her anywheres. Leo's gonna kill me."

Her fear was palpable. I didn't know who Sissy was, but, if a child was missing, I'd need to get the information for a state police AMBER Alert.

"Who's Sissy?" I asked.

Zee's head was down, so I could barely hear her when she answered.

"My python. Well, she's really Leo's and…"

When you've done this as long as I, you think you've heard everything, but, of course, given the creative and perverse nature of human beings, that would be impossible, since people have an infinite capacity for creating an infinite number of circumstances in their lives that defy anyone else's ability to imagine. So, after years of hearing thousands of variations on the human condition, I admit, very occasionally, when a client is talking, I listen with one ear—until Zee said "…and I don't even have any money for rats…"

That phrase caught my attention.

"Rats? Why do you need rats?"

She looked at me like I was stupid.

With barely contained exasperation, she said, "I need to buy a rat to put in Sissy's cage so, when she smells the rat, she'll come out 'cause she's hungry, and Leo won't find out I lost her."

Zee's priority was finding her boyfriend's lost python, while I was stuck knowing that, when Zee delivered, her baby would test positive for alcohol and heroin and would eventually be diagnosed as learning disabled or special needs.

How could I be so sure? If you drop a worm in a glass of gin, it shrivels up and dies. What d'you think happens when the fetal brain is marinated in alcohol for nine months? There was a very high probability Zee's little baby was already brain-damaged, and there wasn't a damn thing I could do about it.

From the day Zee told me she was pregnant, I tried everything I could think of to get her to go into residential treatment. I arranged to get her an ultrasound hoping that, if she could see it, she'd bond with her baby. When the ultrasound suggested she was going to have a girl, Zee told me she was going to name the baby Zoey. "Just like me," she said, "Zoey'll be a little Zee, too." But she didn't agree to come in to stay.

I told her her baby might be born with mental retardation. I referred her to inpatient drug treatment for addiction to alcohol and drugs. She skipped all those appointments.

"Because," she said, "Leo, he don't want me talking to those people."

I felt driven to do whatever I could to try to spare Zee and her baby.

It's hard enough trying to get a teenager to do anything. Trying to get an eighteen-year-old addict who has a long trauma history to listen to reason is almost impossible, because the addiction runs everything. But still, I hoped maybe this time I could convince her to come into the shelter so they could take care of her and the baby before any more damage was done. I decided to try one more time. Leaning forward, in as gentle a voice as I could muster, I asked, "Are you ready to go to the Oaks to stay?"

Zee was biting the edge of her cuticle. It was bleeding.

"No! I gotta get a rat before Leo gets home." She wiped her nose with the back of her hand. I handed her a tissue.

After a long pause, I sighed. "How much does a rat cost?"

"Five dollars," she said.

Picturing a snake as fat as a fire hose made me feel like puking.

But, against my better judgment and all ethical practice, I offered Zee a deal. We'd go to the pet store, and I'd buy a rat. Zee could drop it off at their apartment, and then I'd bring her back to the shelter.

Don't get me wrong. I love animals: cats, dogs, birds, bats, bugs, spiders, toads, okay. But snakes? Yeah, yeah, I know...not slimy, usually not poisonous, good for the environment, yadda, yadda, yadda. What can I say? I'm phobic. I did have some reservations about the whole rat vs. snake issue, but, for me, babies trump everything. I knew very well that what I was offering was wrong. But I couldn't stand the thought that I hadn't done everything I could think of to spare the baby.

Zee shook her head no. "I gotta go," she said. She walked out of the office and slammed the door behind her.

For a second, I almost went after her but stopped myself. Even if I did manage to do the whole buy-the-rat thing, there wasn't any chance that Zee would keep her word and enter residential treatment. The addiction runs everything. Couple that with the power of Leo, and it's game over.

The rest of the story

The next week, I heard through the grapevine that Zee was once again arrested, and, this time, as part of her sentence, the judge ordered her to inpatient treatment. About four months later, Zee showed up at the clinic, carrying an infant in a baby carrier.

"Mizz B, I want you to see the baby. We named him Jesus," or, as she pronounced it, Hay-zeus, "because he is a blessing from God."

All I could think at that moment was that, like everything else about this situation, even the ultrasound was wrong.

I looked down and saw a gorgeous little boy and also saw the telltale signs of a baby with Fetal Alcohol Syndrome. His beautiful, brown eyes were smaller than usual and had epicanthic folds in the corners. His philtrum, the little dent between the top lip and his nose, was totally flat, no dent. My great-grandmother used to say that little dent was where the angels blessed you before you left heaven. The margins of his lips were almost invisible. His ears were set very low on his head. My heart sank. But what was I going to say? Nothing, except, "He's beautiful."

Time would bring its own experiences. Jesus would face challenges all his life, but, with luck, he might be one of the lucky few with FAS who somehow develop great artistic or musical skills. I silently prayed my best prayer: *God, please help him*. I thanked Zee for bringing the baby and asked how she was doing.

"I'm good. Me and Leo are getting ready to take Jesus and go to Mexico."

14

LADY GODIVA

Monday morning, 8:35 a.m.

Before I could take my first sip of coffee, Hannah Legget, my clinic supervisor, called. "Hey, I need you to go over to the crisis unit and do an assessment on a woman they Baker Acted last night. It's Simka Jacklin." (In Florida, the Baker Act allows for what some call emergency or involuntary commitment. It can be initiated by judges, law enforcement officials, physicians, or mental health professionals. There must be evidence that the person possibly has a mental illness.)

Simka Jacklin was in our crisis unit—Simka Jacklin, the Pulitzer Prize-winning author. It was like hearing a unicorn was grazing in the parking lot. I walked across the courtyard to the crisis unit and buzzed the bell. As soon as Matt, a unit aide, unlocked the door, I heard a high-pitched wail rolling down the green-tiled hallway.

"*Goddamned motherf--kers, let me outtt, let me outtt, lemmeow... lemmeoww, lemmeowww...*"

I looked at Matt. "Ms. Jacklin?"

"Yeah, Dr. Sydney gave her a load of Thorazine this morning, but..."

I stopped at the nurse's station to look at Ms. Jacklin's chart, scanned the intake info then the police report.

> Palmetto County Sherriff
> Location: Palmetto Center Highway
> 10-27-1994
> 12:43 a.m.
>
> Subject was seen by this officer, running down the centerline of Cypress Highway. Subject was naked and shouting at passing cars. Officer Gaines halted traffic and attempted to approach subject who ran toward this officer, screaming. Subject was ordered to stop; subject did not comply. Subject was incoherent and attempted to kick and slap Officer Gaines. It was necessary to use reasonable force to restrain her. Subject was unable or willing to identify herself. We attempted to cover her with a sheet, but that was not successful. Subject continued to scream incoherently. Subject was transported to Palmetto County Hospital for a mental health assessment. Dr. Carter Macowen signed a three-day Baker Act for involuntary commitment, and Ms. Jacklin was transported to the Crisis Unit at Palmetto Behavioral Health Clinic.

I put the chart down on the intake desk and looked at May Shepherd, the duty nurse, who was busy updating charts. May was smart, looked like Farrah Fawcett, and was a truly good person. We were lucky to have her on staff.

"When's Dr. Sydney coming back?"

"We've already called him. As soon as he finishes an eval at the jail, he'll be back. Polly Carr's doing the 24/7 observation on her."

"Thanks. I'm going down to take a look-see."

"Good luck with that."

As I approached the observation room, the wailing bounced off the tiled walls and drilled through my head like a car alarm.

"Lemmmeeeowwwww..."

Polly Carr, 30-ish, another unit aide, was sitting on a metal, folding chair outside the room, leafing through a magazine. That morning, she was wearing one of her more bohemian outfits: a gauzy, peasant blouse; swishy, paisley skirt; and huge, gold hoop earrings. Polly was one of the calmest people I've ever met which made her perfect for the job of monitoring Simka Jacklin.

"Hey, Poll, how're we doing?"

"She's got a lot of stamina, I'll say that. Dr. Sydney came by early and gave her 100 mgs. of Thorazine. She calmed down for a little while, but she's still spinning."

Ms. Jacklin popped up behind the observation window and slapped the door so hard I jumped. Smushing her face against the window, she screamed, "I. Am. A. Star. Get me *ooouuuttt of here... get me ooouuuttt of here.*" Her wild, red hair, snarled like a bird's nest, made her look like an enraged Muppet.

Then she backed up, bent over, and mooned me. "Kiss my a--."

Okay. Simka Jacklin was in a full manic mode. Until Sol Sydney got back and adjusted the meds, the best we could do was to keep her safe.

"Poll, let me know when she calms down." I turned to leave, then stopped, because I believe there's always just one more thing to try to reach the person inside their symptoms. I peered through the observation window.

Simka now lay curled in a fetal position, sucking her thumb. I signaled Polly to unlock the door but to stand by. Simka heard the lock click and leaped to her feet. In the universally understood signal for be quiet, I put my forefinger to my lips and stood in the doorway, as if listening for something.

After all the screaming, I figured she must be thirsty. I decided to appeal to her I. Am. A. Star. persona.

"Ms. Jacklin," I whispered, "I wondered if you wanted your juice now or later?"

She furrowed her brow. "Juice?"

"Well, yes, I thought you might be thirsty."

Frozen in indecision, she hesitated.

"Ms. Jacklin?"

Channeling Norma Desmond in *Sunset Boulevard*, she said, "Orange juice—no pulp," then sashayed over to the bed and waved me off to fetch her juice.

I stepped outside the door. Polly locked it.

"Orange juice—no pulp," Polly mimicked.

"Hey, whatever works."

Back at the nurses' station, I asked May, "D'you have any orange juice on hand?"

"We do. Take a look in the unit fridge."

Sure enough, there were about a dozen small cans of OJ in there. I could just imagine what kind of reception canned OJ was going to make on Ms. I. Am. A. Star. I spotted a small wicker tray on the windowsill in the staff break room.

I poured the juice into a flimsy plastic cup and put it on the tray. Outside the observation room, I whispered to Polly, "Knock on the door and say 'Room service.'"

Polly knocked. "Room service."

Simka appeared at the window and stepped back. "Come."

Polly unlocked the door. I bowed my head and proffered the tray. At first, it might seem like a strange tactic to adopt the guise of a server, but, in fact, I think it was a way to subconsciously give Simka the homage she felt she deserved. In "therapy" language, it's called taking a one-down position, my own version of *She Stoops to Conquer*.

One might question the wisdom of allying with a patient's delusion—i.e., she is a star who has been thwarted in her starring role. There are many professionals who would see my offering a client a cup of juice in the guise of being a room service waiter as either unprofessional, enabling, or a breach of boundaries. So, should I just turn my back and let her rave, or try to offer her a cold drink, something that might give her a sense of contact and comfort? No contest.

"Ms. Jacklin?" I proffered the juice. She lifted the juice off the tray, took a sip, then downed the whole thing in a few gulps. I held out the tray for her to replace the cup. "May I get you anything else?"

"Yes...get me outtt of heeere."

Apparently, the contact and comfort thing wasn't working. Holding the tray like a shield, I squeezed out the door Polly was holding open. The lock clicked shut just as Simka hit the door. She smushed her face against the window. *"Getttmeeeoutofheeere..."*

Polly, eyebrows raised and a tiny smile, looked at me.

"Okay, at least I tried. Guess we'll have to wait for Sol to get back." An hour later, Sol Sydney arrived. Simka was still going strong. I wondered if maybe the OJ had helped recharge her batteries, but, given the severity of this episode, one small glass of juice couldn't have had any effect on her mood; might as well throw a cup of water into the ocean and expect it to rise.

Sol looked at me. "Hmmm. I thought the Thorazine would have slowed her down. I'm gonna up her dosage." He went back to the nursing station where the meds were stored.

He returned, followed by Wade. To say Wade was the biggest aide on the unit would be an understatement; he was as big as a queen-sized mattress. The doctor nodded to Polly to open the door.

"Ms. Jacklin? I'm Dr. Sydney. I want to give you something that'll make you feel better."

"I know who the f--k you are. *I feel fine. Get me out of here.*"

Simka wasn't in any mood to talk. Wade stepped into the room. A native of Samoa, he'd been a semi-pro linebacker, but a late hit had ended his career. Because of his size, few people, even in the grip of a psychiatric cyclone, ever really challenged him. His soft-spoken demeanor was the perfect complement to his size.

"Ma'am?" he asked in almost a whisper, "Can you sit down so the doctor can talk to you?"

"He can f--kin' talk to me standin' up."

Wade stepped back, cocked his head, and pointed to the bed. "Ma'am, go ahead and take a seat. You look tired."

Simka stood her ground. Sol and I stood leaning in the open doorway.

Wade gestured with his head toward the bed and said, "Go ahead...rest."

Simka sucked her teeth, whirled around, and sat down on the bed.

"Well?" She looked at Sol. "What the hell do you want?"

"I want to see if we can help you feel better." He gently took her arm and swabbed it. "I hear you're a writer..." He began talking in a soft monotone. Simka sat staring at him as if she were in a trance. Sol Sydney was, in addition to being a great shrink, well versed in hypnotic technique. So, while he didn't perform a formal trance induction, he was able to pace his speech and words in such a soothing way that Simka couldn't help but relax. He slipped the needle into the crook of her elbow and sat murmuring quietly while Wade and I stood against the wall. Imperceptibly, I saw Simka's body lose some tension. Her eye blink slowed. Between the meds and Sol's magic, it looked like Simka was coming out of the storm. She lay down, closing her eyes.

There are some who will take deep umbrage that Simka was medicated without her express consent. There is an ongoing debate about the practice of medicating someone who is unwilling or unable to make decisions in his or her own best interest, and, in some states, it is no longer legal to medicate someone without his or her consent.

Back then, it was seen as an act of mercy to give medication to someone who was in the grip of an illness that made rational decision-making impossible. And, for some, bipolar disorder is fatal—one in ten commits suicide. So, getting the illness under control is, in my book, a lifesaving intervention. However, after the high wears off, a fast spiral down isn't uncommon, which is why, before he left that day, Dr. Sydney put Simka on a 24/7, fifteen-minute suicide watch.

"I'm on call tonight; call me and let me know how she's doing."

Wednesday, 3:00 p.m.

Simka Jacklin spent most of Monday sleeping. I stopped in briefly on Monday, and, by Tuesday, it seemed as if she'd re-entered the real world but was still foggy. On Wednesday morning, I walked down the hall, and Matt unlocked the door to the small, private room that was now Simka's new domain. I stood in the doorway. She wore sweatpants and a faded top, clearly unit clothing. Her hair was dull, and she looked like a sad little balloon left behind when the party ended. I reintroduced myself.

"Ms. Jacklin, I'm Pinny, one of the clinicians for the unit."

Head bowed, she sat slumped on the bed and didn't respond.

My heart went out to her. Here was a woman about my age, a Pulitzer Prize winner, locked in a psych unit, wearing castoffs. I pulled the straight-back chair by the table near to the bed.

"Ms. Jacklin? Do you know where you are?" That might sound like a stupid question, but, frequently when a person has been swept up in a manic episode, they don't know why they're locked up.

I once had another client who had a bipolar disorder similar to Simka Jacklin's. One day, in the grip of an episode, he cleaned out his life savings from his bank account and bought four random houses for cash. His wife was frantic, and it wasn't until the police picked him up for a DUI that she caught up with him and found out they were now essentially penniless. It took some fancy and expensive lawyering to undo the deals. The husband, when I first interviewed him, denied he'd done anything wrong and, in fact, had no memory of the house-buying binge. Police reports and financial statements from his wife were testament to his behavior. Once lucid, he was appalled and went into a deep depression, a not-unusual sequence of emotions following a severe manic episode.

Simka continued to stare at the floor but answered my question. "In the psych ward."

"Do you remember how you got here?"

"The police?"

"Do you remember why they brought you here?"

She shook her head slowly side to side.

"Have you been hospitalized before?"

She nodded. "About six years ago, before we moved here from Connecticut. I was in The Institute of Living in Hartford. I have bipolar disorder."

"Was that your first hospitalization?"

"Yes. After my book came out, I couldn't sleep and..." She sounded totally exhausted. It wasn't necessary at that moment to push her. I decided to ask about her history when her husband arrived. After two more days, Simka was discharged from the crisis unit. Her husband took her home, but she returned for a follow-up appointment. I met with her in my office.

"Simka, I've read your chart. You were taking lithium for several years. What made you decide to stop taking it? Were you having side effects?"

"You mean like the fact I gained 30 pounds, felt like a fat pig, and my hands shook all the time?" Sarcasm dripped from her tongue.

I actually sympathized with her. Weight gain is one of the unfortunate side effects of taking lithium; it's literally a big price to pay for stabilizing mood.

Two main reasons why most people who are bipolar decide to stop taking their meds? Virtually all of my bipolar clients reported, at one time or other, the same thing: weight gain and the feeling they just weren't up to par either mentally or energy-wise.

"I hear you. It's a tricky med to manage. But you've been on it a long time; what was going on that made you decide at this particular time that you wanted to stop taking your meds?"

"Okay, I'll tell you." She hesitated. "Okay. I was listening to a Swami somebody or other being interviewed on the radio. He was talking about natural herbs they use in India to control bipolar. Basically, he was saying the reason people get sick is they are in poor health and that Ayurvedic herbs heal the body from within. He talked about regular drugs just healing symptoms, but, once the body is healed by natural herbs, the sickness goes away. It sounds stupid now, but..." She sighed. "I just wanted to see if there was something else I could take that wouldn't make me feel fat and stupid." Tears filled her eyes and spilled over. She reached for a handful of tissues.

"Do you mind if I ask where you got the herbs?"

Her head was bowed, so it was hard to hear her answer. "In the mail."

She didn't need to hear anything from me about staying on her medication. I wrote myself a note to talk to Sol Sydney about what other ideas he might have about treating her depression.

Simka Jacklin was a brilliant woman who'd acquired self-awareness in a most painful way. She was mortified and filled with remorse. "How could I be so stupid?"

"If it helps any, I must tell you that virtually everyone I've seen that has a bipolar disorder has stopped taking their meds for one reason or another. Who can blame them?

"I'm not sure if you've ever heard of her, but there's a doctor who's written extensively about her own experience of living with bipolar disorder, particularly how it affects and relates to creativity. Her name is Dr. Kay Redfield Jamison and her latest book is called *The Fire Within*. Can I suggest you buy it and read it? She's almost as good a writer as you, and she tells, in ways I never could, how to live well despite bipolar disorder...or maybe in concert with it. In any case, I think you might find some of what you're looking for in her book."

Her husband spoke up. "We're stopping at Barnes and Noble on the way home."

Simka looked small and tired.

"Have you made a follow-up appointment with Dr. Sydney?"

"They made it at discharge."

"If you're getting your meds through our clinic, you have to have some regular appointments with a therapist, so I'd like to see you once you've gotten back on your meds. Let's go up to the front desk and make our appointment. When you come back, you can tell me what you think of the book."

The rest of the story

Simka Jacklin returned faithfully for her follow-up appointments. And we did, indeed, talk many times about Dr. Jamison's book. If you're curious about bipolar disorder, pick up any one of Dr. Redfield's books. They're evocative, powerful, and the best source of information on the subject that I've ever read.

15

TIGER, TIGER BURNING BRIGHT

By four o'clock, I'd already seen five clients. As I was finishing my notes on my last session, my phone rang. It was Peg.

"Your four o'clock is here."

I skimmed the intake sheet. Svetlana Nureyva. Seventy-three-year-old woman reports depression related to history of chronic pain. New to the area. Divorced three times. What caught my attention was her address—Ochopee, a tiny town located in the Everglades, most noted for having the smallest post office in the US and being home to the Skunk Ape Research Headquarters.

I was running out of steam. Needing to fortify myself, I opened my desk drawer, unwrapped a bite-sized Milky Way, popped it in my mouth, and went to fetch Ms. Nureyva.

I reached the entrance to the waiting room and was stunned to see the clients down on their knees, bunched in a tight circle, like they were praying to Mecca. An ungodly caterwauling rose from the center of the circle. I almost choked on my Milky Way when I saw what was causing the racket. A pair of twin tiger cubs, no bigger than housecats, were yowling and growling as they wrestled on the floor. Just as one of the clients reached out to touch a cub, a woman, whom I hadn't noticed, stepped into the circle.

"Do not touch them," she said.

Apparently, she'd been standing in the corner watching the small circus she'd brought with her. I walked across the room and introduced myself.

"Ms. Nureyva?" I said. She nodded.

"I'm Pinny Bugaeff. Let's go to my office."

She snapped her fingers at the baby tigers. "Come," she said. The cubs immediately stopped wrestling and padded behind us as I led the way down the hall. I closed the door and nodded toward the wing chair across from my desk. Svetlana, with the grace of a ballerina, sat down and pointed at the larger cub who was trying to climb up her leg.

"That is Boris. I named him after my third husband. And that," she said, pointing to the smaller cub that was hiding behind my plant stand, "is Natasha. They are brother and sister."

Every therapist I know carries on a dual conversation while they're with a client. The first conversation is what we say out loud; the second is what we're thinking but don't say. In this case, I had to restrain myself from saying, "Since Boris and Natasha are here, did you bring Rocky or Bullwinkle?" but, even if we'd already established some kind of therapeutic relationship, that would've been inappropriate. I tend to get a little silly when I'm tired. I tore myself away from watching the cubs.

"Ms. Nureyva," I said.

She interrupted. "Svetlana. Please call me Svetlana."

"Svetlana. Please call me Pinny."

She leaned forward and offered a handshake. Her hand was covered with scars, but before I asked about them, I wanted to give Svetlana a chance to feel more comfortable with me. I sidestepped the scars and opted for small talk.

"Svetlana. I see you're new to the area. Where did you live before you moved to Ochopee?"

"Gibsonton."

She lowered her head, cocked an eyebrow, and looked at me. It felt like I was being tested. If I knew what was significant about

Gibsonton, I'd pass the "Can I trust you test?" that most clients give when they're trying to decide if they want to reveal their deepest secrets to a stranger. Luckily for me, I knew Gibsonton was a small town near Tampa, mostly populated by circus and carnival workers. Town ordinances there allow residents to keep tiger cages and elephants in their yards.

I nodded and smiled encouragement. "I do know about Gibsonton," I said. "Did you know the Lobster Boy?"

Svetlana looked surprised. Lobster Boy's real name was Grady Stiles. In 1992, his wife and stepson were tried for murdering him. Grady had been born with a condition called Ectrodactyly, a birth defect that left him with fingers and feet fused in a way that made them look like lobster claws. At age seven or eight, he began traveling with a carnival sideshow. In his later years, he retired to Gibsonton, where he developed a reputation for having a terrible temper. The trial the year before had been big news, and I'd followed it with the perverse interest that kind of thing engenders in me.

"I did know him," she said. "He vas mean sonoffabeach." Svetlana relaxed and settled back into the chair. Even the heavy makeup she wore couldn't hide the scars that began at her neck and then disappeared beneath the long-sleeved, black top she was wearing. She bent down and picked up Natasha who settled into her lap. Sitting there stroking the cub, she looked like a very old child holding a stuffed animal.

"Svetlana, our initial intake sheet mentioned you have a history of depression and chronic pain." As gently as I could, I asked, "Are the scars related to those things?"

She nodded slowly several times. We sat in silence. I waited for her to tell me her story in her own time.

"So," she said, "the scars...I was in a fire...many people don't know but, in 1961, there was a circus tent fire in Brazil, like the one in Hartford. And when the tent was burning...I tried to help them...the children..." Her voice broke.

I'd read a book about the 1944 Ringling Brothers fire. The tent had been treated with paraffin and gasoline to waterproof it. It caught fire and burned to the ground. Hundreds died. Many suffered terrible burns. I later looked up the fire in Brazil. It was almost a virtual replay of the Hartford fire.

"The cages...they blocked the doors..." she continued. "I try but...I only got out one little girl." She raised her hands, palms up, wordlessly saying, "What could I do?" Tears ran down her cheeks. I watched her stroking the little tiger that slept in her lap.

"That is why I need medicine. I had doctor when I lived in Tampa, but now I am here, I need medicine for my pain and...I still have dreams." She reached for a tissue.

Just then, Boris arched his butt and peed on the carpet.

"*Boris!*" Svetlana yelled and jumped out of the chair. Looking pleased with himself, Boris rolled over on his back.

"I am so sorry," Svetlana said. She reached for the box of tissues, knelt down, and tried to swab up the rank puddle of tiger pee.

Actually, I wasn't concerned. It was a dark brown, industrial carpet. What's a little tiger pee? Besides, Boris had done me a favor. Svetlana was about to plunge back into the fires of hell, but it was 4:45 p.m., almost time for the session to end, not the right time to rekindle smoldering memories. I stood, went around the desk, knelt down next to Svetlana, and grabbed a handful of tissues. Svetlana stopped her scrubbing and looked over at me like she expected me to be angry.

"I've diapered babies and shoveled horse manure," I said, "but this is my first time for tiger pee." I was laughing.

Boris rolled over and batted her arm. "Oh, you are a very bad boy," she said.

"Kids...what can you do?" I said. She smiled.

The rest of the story

After several more sessions with Svetlana, I felt she needed intensive trauma treatment that was beyond my level of expertise.

Having greatly benefitted from treatment with hypnotherapy for my own PTSD issues, I referred Svetlana for treatment to a local psychiatrist who was a friend and well versed in that modality. I also made a referral to a pain management clinic. Although I never saw Svetlana again, when I saw my friend the psychiatrist, he thanked me for sending him such an interesting person and told me my tiger lady was doing well. He also told me she was now the mother of a lion cub and two cheetahs.

Over the next two years, on very humid days, the faint scent of tiger pee reminded me how blessed I was to be doing the work I loved.

16

WE'RE BAAAAACK

After eleven years in Florida, Alex and I had rebuilt our lives. We were happy. Our son, Gregor, had moved to Fort Lauderdale and joined the art scene there. Mandy, who still lived in Connecticut, married Mark, a guy we were crazy about. A few years later, they announced she was pregnant. I knew I'd love being a grandmother, but, at that moment, I didn't realize just what an impact that baby would have on us.

We got the call from Mark that Mandy was in labor, and we flew back to Connecticut in time for the birth. I couldn't have imagined a lovelier bonding experience of waiting through a long night of labor with the two other sets of grands, then sharing the joy of the birth of our eight-pound nine-ounce granddaughter, Hannah Katherine.

To say it was hard for us to get back on the plane and leave Mandy, Mark, and the baby was an understatement. Three months later, Mandy called and said she'd like to come down with the baby for a visit. We were over the moon.

All the time they were with us, I was practically velcroed to baby Hannah. Being a mother is an amazing and daunting experience. Being a grandmother—pure bliss. The two-week visit flew by. With heavy hearts, we took Mandy and Hannah to the airport and watched their plane taxi down the runway, taking them back to Connecticut. I cried all the way home. Alex was quiet.

Back at the house, I sat on the couch and couldn't stop crying. Alex sat down and put his arm around me.

"I can't live this far away from them," I sobbed. He took a deep breath.

"You wouldn't think of moving back to Connecticut…would you?" He sounded incredulous.

"Yes," I sobbed.

He took another deep breath. "Me too," he said, and then we were laughing.

The magnetic force of a tiny baby drew us out of Florida and back to Connecticut. It took a whole year for us to sell the house and for both of us to get new jobs in New England, but we did it. Alex was hired by a tech company, and I was hired as a clinician to work in a halfway house for female offenders.

The next five years brought us the birth of Hannah's brother, Atticus. If I thought one grandbaby filled my heart to overflowing, I discovered the heart expands to hold enough love for however many more the universe decides to send.

My brother, Peter, died at age 44, and my sister-in-law died soon after, so, when their daughter, Kim, had a beautiful baby girl, whom they named Eva, and, when my nephew and his wife had twins, whom they named Finn and Sydney, I became their honorary grandmother.

So, in total, I'm blessed with five grands. We never looked back, never questioned our decision to leave our Gulf Coast paradise. Love and babies have kept us warm, even through the coldest winters. Working with the women who came through the program at the halfway house was, to say the least, an education.

17

TELL ME A STORY

I pulled into the parking lot of the halfway house to begin my three-to-eleven shift. Two months into the job and I was already tired. Dealing with fifteen women, all of whom had trauma histories and multiple issues with the legal system, was challenging to say the least. Thunder rolled in the distance. Fat raindrops splatted my windshield. I hurried up the steps of the dilapidated, Victorian house that was Stone Haven. When I opened the front door, the smell of fish frying nearly knocked me over. Hip-hop music pulsed through the air, almost drowning out the roar of the vacuum Charlene was dragging down the hall. The cacophony drove me out to the back porch. It was raining hard.

I WAS SIX AGAIN, RUNNING THROUGH THE RAIN, AWAY FROM MY brother, Peter, who was bellowing threats of mayhem as he chased me out of the house because I'd accidently stepped on his model plane. After running two blocks, my six-year-old legs were getting tired. Desperate for sanctuary, I darted across a busy street and flew up the steps of a huge, granite building.

Heart pounding, gasping for breath, I burst into the lobby of the Carnegie Library and skidded up to the mahogany checkout desk. A librarian pointed to French doors just beyond the desk and whispered, "The children's room is over there."

Like a cartoon bum lured by the smell of an apple pie cooling on a windowsill, I opened the French doors and stepped in. Dust motes hung like filmy curtains in front of the gothic windows. Little tables were laid out with books. While I caught my breath, I circled the tables. One book cover caught my eye—a young boy, dressed in a red tunic, stood looking out to sea; black storm clouds hovered over him; fish were leaping helter-skelter behind him—*Leif the Lucky.*

I quietly pulled out a chair, opened the book, and sailed away with Leif on his Viking ship. We landed in Greenland, but howling Skraelings chased us back to our longboats. The library lights flicked off and on. It was starting to get dark outside. A lady in a plaid skirt came over to my little table and pointed to the book.

"Would you like to take that book home with you?"

Although I knew libraries had lots of books to read, surely, they wouldn't let a six-year-old just walk out with a beautiful book. And besides, everyone knew you had to pay for something before you took it out of a store. I thought maybe the library lady was pulling a prank on me. I was no dummy. I looked at her with whatever could pass for a jaundiced eye in a six-year-old.

"Would you like to take it home? You know all you have to do is sign your name on a card, and you can borrow it for two weeks."

There had to be a catch.

"Can you write your name?"

I nodded.

"Do you know your street address and telephone number?"

I nodded.

"Well, that's all you need to borrow a book. If you come over to the desk, I'll show you how." Still suspicious, I followed her to see just how long she was going to keep up the farce. Once behind the desk, she handed me a white card with lines for name, address, and phone number.

"Just fill those in, and you can have a library card."

In wobbly, first-grade letters, I printed my name, address, and phone number. The librarian looked at the card and put it into a file box. Then she took *Leif the Lucky*, opened it to the back cover, took out the card, stamped another card, and slid it into a little paper pocket glued to the inside back cover. She handed me a small, tan card with my name on it. "Here's your library card," she said, and pushed the book across the desk to me. "Just bring the book back in two weeks." She looked at the calendar. "That's on April tenth." I figured I'd remember, since it was my birthday. "When you bring one back, you can then take out four more."

Okay, now I knew she was lying. Who's going to give a six-year-old four books to take home and believes the kid'll bring them back? It was getting darker outside. I was already in trouble for my brother's stupid broken plane. If I didn't get home soon, I'd be in my room with no supper.

Clutching *Leif* with one hand, I ran all the way home. I knew nobody would believe me if I said they let me into the library and a nice lady told me to take the book home for free, so I hid it under the bench on the porch.

Later, after everyone was asleep, I sneaked downstairs and brought the book up to my room. Scrunched in my closet with my flashlight, I once more set sail for Greenland.

Two weeks later was Saturday, my birthday. I put on a sweatshirt, stuck the book underneath it, and hoped nobody would see me crossing Watchung Avenue.

I ran up the steps of the library but stopped short in the lobby. Hanging just behind the checkout desk was a life-sized painting of two beautiful women. They stood on a cliff above the sea, watching for someone. I imagined they were watching for me. Slipping past the main desk, I opened the doors to the children's room. I hoped the nice lady was there, because I wasn't 100 percent sure this taking-books-out deal was kosher. I pulled the *Leif* book from under my sweatshirt and put it on the desk.

"Oh, you're right on time," the lady said and pulled the card from the back of the book.

On days when there were other kids in the library, the lady in the plaid skirt, whose name was Miss Hallow, would invite us to story circle. She read to us using an amazing variety of wonderful voices that made the story come alive. On days when there were no other kids around, she'd still come over and ask me if I'd like to come to story circle, and she'd read a story just for me. I was almost eight before I figured out Miss Hallow designated story circle to coincide with whatever time I might show up.

Safe inside the bastion of books, I listened and learned. Leif the Lucky sailed away on his own, the Ugly Duckling finally found her family, and wicked witches could be foiled.

I SIGHED AT THE MEMORY AND DRAGGED MYSELF BACK FROM THE PAST to the Stone Haven porch. It was still raining. Listening to the chaos inside, I was dreading the group I was supposed to run that night. Two groups a week for the past two months, and not much had changed since the first night we met. The first group went like this:

"Tonight, we're going to introduce ourselves and say a little about what you hope to get out of group. My name is Pinny Bugaeff. I'm a social worker, and I've just moved here. Tonight, I'd just like to talk with you, and maybe together we can help you figure out what you want to do when you're back in the community. First, I'd like to go around the circle, tell me your name and what you hope to get out of this group." I nodded at the woman across from me, indicating she could start.

"Charlene," she said, then sat there breathing through her mouth.

OK, maybe she's a little slow.

"What brought you here, Charlene?"

A few of the women rolled their eyes at my question.

"The big bus," she said.

I caught the women smirking at each other. I shifted my focus to the skinny woman sitting to the right of Charlene. She looked terminally bored. I tried nodding and smiling at her to indicate it was her turn.

She mumbled, "Sharone." That was it.

The next two ladies, Tessa and Chyna, were more forthcoming. Tessa talked about how much she missed her children. She was 27, had six kids, and earnestly believed selling crack had been a good job for a stay-at-home mom.

Chyna had one thing on her mind. "I'm getting a job and saving up, and, when I get out, I'm going to go as far away from here as I can get."

The woman sitting next to Chyna sat in sullen silence, her massive arms crossed over her chest. The scar at her hairline slashed diagonally across her face, leaving a visage Picasso would have loved. I thought if I could find my way into helping her, maybe God would erase one line of my sins from His books. I smiled at her.

"You are...?"

"Janeese," she said, pronouncing her name as though it began with a French J. "I sure do hope to get out of this group."

Everybody laughed and bumped fists. I ignored her comment. She sat through the rest of the session staring at a spot slightly to the right of my ear, aimlessly picking at the needle scars that pocked her arms. I wondered what I might do to breach her wall of rage. Nothing came to mind.

We sat in silence until Tessa asked, "How come I can't go home on a pass this week?"

Chyna snapped, "Bitch, you're on restriction!"

In an attempt to get somebody to talk to me, I asked them to tell me about restrictions. The remaining ten minutes of that first group were spent trying to understand what led to Tessa's restriction and why she didn't deserve it. The next two sessions weren't much better.

Standing on the porch, listening to the rain, I thought, *Trying to do therapy with this bunch is like trying to turn toasters into TVs.* Then I remembered. I'd bought a Little Golden Book for Hannah that day. I went into my office and rummaged through my purse until I found it. *The Ugly Duckling.*

At seven o'clock, the ladies ambled into the group room. I asked Tessa to open the windows. A rain-scented breeze rippled the curtains. I flipped off the overhead light, pulled my chair close to the table lamp, and opened the book.

"Once upon a time…"

Janeese snorted, "This ain't group."

Ignoring her, I continued, "…a little duck…"

Janeese sucked her teeth. "A duck?"

I continued to read. Quiet settled over the circle. I glanced up to see how the women were responding to being read a kiddies' book. They were entranced. I continued through to the end. "…and the Ugly Duckling grew into a beautiful swan and flew gracefully into the sky to join the flock on their long journey." I closed the book and waited.

Finally, Sharone broke the silence. Staring at the floor, she said, "I'm a lot darker than my sisters."

While we sat listening to Sharone tell her story of isolation and pain, I was thinking about how the Ugly Duckling had waddled through Sharone's defenses. However, Janeese was thinking about food. "It's snack time," she growled. The group broke up.

I read *Beauty and the Beast* to my next story circle, which led to a hot discussion about the men in their lives. At the end of group, I asked them each to write a one-page story about why they thought Beauty stayed with the Beast. They would be the storytellers for the next group.

Two weeks later, I read them *Snow White and the Seven Dwarfs*. At the end of the story, Charlene raised her hand. I nodded to her, encouraging her to share. Although I listened patiently while she told a rambling and graphic story about a well-paid weekend she'd spent in Las Vegas with twin brothers who owned a casino off the strip, I was puzzled.

"Why did the Snow White story remind you of the twins in Las Vegas?"

She replied, "…de was doorfs."

I had a special place in my heart for Charlene. Like most of the women in the halfway house, she was a victim of abuse and had problems with addictions. And, like most, she'd had an unspeakable childhood. One afternoon, I saw her sitting by herself on the picnic bench in the yard. She was wearing a tank top and shorts. I went outside and sat down next to her, just to visit. It was then I noticed the scars, little white scars—tiny parallel lines crisscrossing her cocoa-brown shoulders. I glanced down and saw hundreds of similar scars on her legs.

She saw me looking. Although Charlene was a little slow, she was pretty smart about reading people.

"Ya lookin' at dees?" She gestured to her shoulder and legs. I nodded.

She said, "mymothahitmewithastechioncor."

I didn't get what she was saying. "Your mother did what?"

"She hit me with a stetchin cor."

I was flummoxed. I didn't want Charlene to be re-traumatized because her therapist couldn't understand her. Gently I asked her, "Charlene, what's a stetchin cor?"

She looked at me like I was slow. "Ya know," she said, "it's one o' those long 'lectric cords ya use to plug in somethin'."

I got it. Charlene's mother had beaten her regularly with an extension cord, and the tiny, white parallel scars were evidence she'd whipped her with the end with the plug. I wondered if Charlene might have been born with a normal intelligence and then maybe, at the hands of her mother, suffered a head injury which had left her now so impaired. I felt sick, angry, and powerless.

That night, I was reading *The Velveteen Rabbit*. I glanced up at the circle of faces and caught four pairs of little-girl eyes peering over the tops of their fortress walls. I continued reading.

"A little brown bunny peeked through the bushes. The Velveteen Rabbit was finally real."

Glancing up again, I saw the women brushing tears from their eyes, except for Janeese, who still sat in sullen silence; unmoved, unmoving.

Everybody scattered to finish their evening chores. Charlene fired up the vacuum. Tessa went to the kitchen and cranked up the radio. I went outside. Janeese was sweeping the porch. She slowly swept her way to where I was standing and leaned her broom against the porch railing.

"I usta' have a bunny," she said. "My daddy killed it."

We stood in the dark, and Janeese began to tell me her story.

Janeese never did share in group, but, after group, she'd come out to the porch. We'd stand side by side, staring into the darkness, and she'd talk about the hellish life she'd endured. She became the storyteller, and I listened with all my heart.

The rest of the story

For 40 years, I dreamed about the library lady, Miss Hallow, and that painting—the one that hung above the checkout desk—two women looking out over the sea, watching for someone.

In 1986, I went to a Winslow Homer art exhibit at the Yale New Haven Gallery. I walked in the door, and there was the painting—two beautiful women on the cliff, still watching. I wanted to tell them that, despite a few shipwrecks and several encounters with Skraelings, I'd made it. I had a home of my own, a husband as brave as a Viking, two beautiful children, amazing grandchildren, friends, and a wonderful life.

Thank you, Miss Hallow, my library angel. Stories saved my life. And partly, because I loved stories, listening to them, and telling them, I became a therapist. I've spent the better part of 40 years listening to the stories of other kids who survived and have done my best to help them write new stories with better endings.

I spent five years working with a bevy of beautiful, wicked, smart, nasty, kind, and funny women. Many took advantage of what the program had to offer. Some didn't. One thing was clear to me. It's far easier to modify behavior, thoughts, and feelings before years of abuse hammer the spirit into a hardened mass of pain.

Five years working the three-to-eleven shift in an environment so full of trauma was starting to wear me down. Although I was taking good care of myself, I was on the verge of experiencing secondary trauma, which happens when a person is exposed to a daily diet of crises and pain. It's a well-known phenomenon in the helping professions, and I recognized it was time for me to find another way to use my skills.

I thought about what drew me into the field to begin with. I remembered the day I walked into the block house at Manida Street. I remembered Phyllis. I remembered how much I liked working with kids. Maybe if I got to the kids and their parents early enough, somewhere down the line, the kids would have a chance. I'd always been lucky finding a job when I needed one, and this time was no exception. After completing an application and reams of paperwork, I was hired as a clinical consultant for a private Children's Services Agency.

18

KID IN A CAGE

One of my duties at Children's Services was to make home visits to families who were fostering children that had special needs for either physical or cognitive challenges. My supervisor asked me to go out and do an assessment of a foster child who'd been placed for a year but didn't seem to be making progress.

Early autumn, I pulled up to a tidy little house located in an older development. I noticed the yard was freshly raked of leaves, and the bushes were neatly trimmed. When I knocked on the door, a woman who looked to be in her late 40s answered. I introduced myself, and she gave me a firm but chilly handshake; not a big deal, a lot of our foster parents didn't welcome the social worker poking into their business.

The first thing I saw when I walked into the living room was a small pet carrier, about the size of a shoe box, sitting on the end shelf of a bookcase. A tiny whimpering came out of the box. I went over and peeked in. A Chihuahua was lying flat on its belly, his pointy little ears touching the inside top of the box. I turned to the foster mother. Clearly, she read the look on my face.

"Oh, I hardly ever put him in there," she said. "I didn't want him getting underfoot while you all were here."

I was there to assess the progress her two-year-old foster child, Bobby, was making, but the situation with the little dog was, to me, not just a red flag, but a waving, giant, crimson banner. Anyone who would confine an animal in a box like the one on the bookcase was immediately suspect in my book, because people tend to treat pets and kids the same. For instance, people who love animals often turn out to be awesome foster parents, because they have high tolerance for pesky behavior, oceans of patience, and love to spare.

In any case, right after I passed the Chihuahua in the shoe box, I followed the foster mother into an immaculate family room. Baby Bobby was holding onto the top rail of a crib, sidestepping slowly around the inside perimeter. He didn't even look up when we entered the room, just slowly slid his left leg forward and dragged his right leg along step by step until he'd managed to circumnavigate the crib.

If you've ever seen an animal in the zoo, pacing the cage, you'll have an idea of what I was seeing. There was mindlessness to his movement that was so apparent it made me feel sick. The baby's hair hung in thin, greasy strands; his eyes had the dullness that's a hallmark of a depressed baby. I went over and knelt down to his level. He didn't look at me, just kept moving around and around. I didn't trust myself to speak. I was so angry, I wanted to grab him up and take him out of there.

Bobby had been born with limited ability to move his right leg, and his coordination was impaired. Because Bobby was a foster child who required a higher level of care than a kid without any neurological problems, I'd taken the time to read through his entire record, starting with his birth records and progressing through a stack of files a foot tall.

The records detailed the extent of Bobby's impairments, his need for specialized care, prescriptions for exercises from a physical therapist and a pediatrician that indicated, that, with proper therapy, his prognosis for being able to gain full function was pretty good. If given regular exercises and therapy, he'd acquire the strength and agility that would likely lead to a life without any restrictions.

Bobby had been placed in foster care as a one-year-old. As I read through the files, I noted that, in prior home visits, several workers had each commented on the fact that Bobby didn't seem to be making much progress with his physical limitations and that, despite strong recommendations from the doctors, Bobby spent a lot of time in a crib the foster mother kept in the family room.

I took some cleansing breaths before I opened a conversation with the foster mother.

"I see that Bobby's in the crib."

"Oh, that was just because you were coming to see him, and I wanted the house to be tidy."

I walked over to the crib, bent down, and picked up the baby.

"Well, how about if we take Mr. Bobby out of the crib, and let's see how he's doing?"

He lay on the floor like a rag doll. After watching him lie there for a minute, I picked him up and gently began to rub his back.

"I took a look at some of the exercises the physical therapist recommended. How's he doing with pulling little sacks of groceries around the kitchen?"

"Well, truthfully, it just takes too long to get the groceries out of the car, then I have to get Bobby in the house, but first I have to put Chi-Chi out of the way." (I assumed Chi-Chi was the Chihuahua.) "Then I have to put the groceries away..." She trailed off.

"Well, how's he doing with sitting on the bouncy ball?" Since there was no big, therapeutic, bouncy ball visible in the room, I was curious to see what she'd say.

"Oh, the bouncy ball. It was so big, and Chi-Chi was always trying to bite it, so I put it in the garage."

"Does Bobby do his ball balance exercises there?" I knew the answer to that. I knew damn well Bobby was no better off than

Chi-Chi. Both spent their days in a pen or a box so that "Mom" could keep the house and yard neat as a pin.

"Well, I try to take him outside every day…"

This "mom" was being paid a hefty fee to care for this little baby who was depressed and still unable to move his right side with anything like fluidity. At that moment, it was all I could do not to just take the baby and leave, or call investigative services, who assess and supervise emergency removals. But this was a tricky case. The house was clean; there was food in the kitchen and no marks I could see on the baby. According to regulations, this wasn't a case of imminent danger.

By now, Bobby had settled against me and was sucking his thumb. It was all I could do to return him to the crib. I wrapped up the conversation as quickly as I could, because I was on a mission to get Bobby out of baby jail.

It was getting dark as I arrived at the main office. I rushed upstairs and began to reread the reports of all the prior home and doctor visits we had on file. Over the previous year, the foster mother had been asked, encouraged, and told directly that she must start implementing the exercises prescribed for Bobby. And yet, here we were a year later, Bobby still spent his days moving around and around and around his tiny prison yard. I wrote up my visit in detail and included very detailed excerpts from previous visits by the doctors and workers, all saying the same thing to the mom. Take the kid out of the cage and let him free range, while you provide interesting and fun exercises that will help him learn to stand and walk and play.

The next morning, I was still on fire. I met briefly with my supervisor and got her to sign off so that I could take the case directly to the supervisor of all children in foster care. I called to alert her. She agreed to read my report. Later the next day, she called me.

"I read your report. We're removing the child today. I have a great family that'll take him." That was it. I didn't care she was terse. I could go home and sleep that night.

I later heard through the grapevine that Bobby was placed with a very experienced couple who'd had good results working with kids with Bobby's physical issues, and they'd applied to adopt him.

Writing this story brought it all back: the anger, the frustration, and the rare sense that, just maybe, I made a difference—at least to one little kid named Bobby.

19

MILO THE SUMO

Prudence, a foster care worker and good friend, asked me to go on a home visit with her, mainly to assess the "fit" between foster parents and Milo, the child they were about to adopt. The little boy was three years old and autistic. The prospective parents were older and had never had children, so there was a question as to whether they were prepared to cope with the issues inherent with a child on the Autism spectrum.

We pulled up to a nice, raised ranch, went to the door, and rang the bell. The mother, a petite brunette maybe in her late 30s, "just call me Barb," invited us in and introduced us to her husband, who was lounging in a recliner wearing a T-shirt and sweatpants. He gave us a nod but wasn't what you'd call cordial. Most prospective parents want to make a good impression on the workers. Nonetheless, I figured maybe he was tired from chasing a three-year-old, or maybe he was just a laid-back kind of guy.

Usually, when I did a home assessment visit, I liked to take a few minutes and watch the dynamics in the home. When Prudence began to talk with the mother, I took a seat on the circular sofa and noticed there was a little bowl of dry Cheerios on the coffee table in front of me. At that point, Milo, who looked like a miniature Michelin Man, came running into the living room. He ran over to the orange cat that was sleeping on the floor in a patch of sun and kicked it, hard. I expected a reaction of some kind from the mother or father.

The mother said in a little, whiny voice, "Milo, don't kick the cat."

Milo, as one might expect, ignored her. It's never a good sign when kids are allowed to abuse the family pets, but I tried to maintain a semblance of professionalism when I turned to the mother and asked, "Is that how you normally handle Milo kicking the cat?"

"Oh," she said, "he doesn't kick the cat that often."

Oh boy—"that often." Her answer confirmed what I'd implied in my question. Milo was a frequent cat kicker.

A minute later, Milo picked up a slipper and threw it at his father in the recliner. I waited to see what would happen.

"Milo," the dad said, without taking his eyes off the TV, "it's not nice to throw shoes."

Mentally, I was trying to give the prospective parents the benefit of the doubt. I thought maybe they were intimidated by our presence and wondered if they'd do differently if they weren't nervous about being observed, but, truthfully, I had my doubts about this whole setup.

Just then, Milo wandered over to the coffee table and stood right next to me. He picked up a Cheerio and popped it in his mouth. I followed suit. I picked up a Cheerio and popped it in my mouth. Milo reached for another Cheerio and put it on the table. I reached for a Cheerio to put on the table. Milo grabbed my arm and bit down so hard I felt the skin burst.

He was tremendously strong and held my arm in a vise-like grip. I yelped and turned sideways, trying to get him into what's called a therapeutic basket hold, but the couch was wedged so close to the enormous coffee table, I couldn't find space to move. The mother just watched me struggling to disengage Milo. The father, glued to the TV, remained in his recliner. I managed to stand up, but Milo clung like a tiger to my arm, torqueing and twisting it until I felt something in my shoulder let go. Prudence ran over and managed to pull Milo away.

I'm not clear what happened next, except I found I couldn't lift my arm above my waist. It wasn't the pain, because I think I was in shock; it just wasn't physically possible to lift my arm. Something was terribly wrong. Prudence took charge, and, with little fuss, we left.

Since it was protocol to immediately report any kind of on-the-job accident, Prudence drove us back to the office and sent me directly to my supervisor. I told her what happened. She gave me a form to fill out and told me I had to go to the agency-contracted walk-in clinic for a preliminary examination. Normally, I'd call my doctor or go to the ER, but that wasn't agency protocol, which, if it wasn't followed, could have invalidated any covered costs incurred from the injury.

I was granted the rest of the day off and drove myself, one armed, to the clinic where I waited an hour to be seen. The bite was swelling, and I still couldn't raise my arm. At 5:00 p.m., I finally saw a doctor. He cleaned the bite and gave me a shot, all the while minimizing my chief complaint, which was that I couldn't raise my arm.

"It's probably sprained; take some Ibuprofen and go see your own doctor if it doesn't feel better."

By the time I got home, my arm was killing me. I called my orthopedist that night and described my symptoms. He told me he'd see me the next morning.

The rest of the story

A week later, I went in for rotator cuff surgery. The damage was so extensive, the repair required three titanium screws and four months of rehab. I had a lot of time to think while I was recuperating. Here I was, age 67, over 40 years working with some very dangerous and volatile clients in some fairly dangerous environments, and never got a scratch, then a three-year-old tears me up.

I was old enough and had lived long enough to know that, when God wants to get my attention, He first gives me a gentle nudge and, if I ignore that, He arranges something that, in the long run, will be to my benefit, but, in the short run…not so much. I'm not saying God sent a three-year-old to terrorize me, but I got the message.

The four months I spent recovering reminded me what it was like to have leisure time; time to see my children and grandchildren, time to daydream, to spend time with Alex, time to cook and read, and, finally, time to begin writing. Work no longer called to me. I wanted to stay home and play but was reluctant to give up the salary.

Alex, Gregor, and Mandy, even my grandchildren, Hannah and Atticus, all said, in their own way: It's okay to stop. One day, I was agonizing to Mandy about my dilemma. Atticus, age seven, was listening.

"Peach," he said, (that was my grandmother name) "why don't you just quit?"

"Well, if I quit, I won't be able to buy you cool presents like helicopters and stuff."

"Peach," he said, standing in front of me, as serious as a seven-year-old can be. "I'd rather have you happy than have cool stuff."

That night, Alex sat down next to me on the couch and hugged me tight.

"You don't have to do this anymore. Quit. The money is nothing. We'll find a way, like we always do."

The next Monday, I went into work and turned in my letter of resignation. After all the paperwork and a retirement party, I discovered that part of my retirement package included health coverage for both Alex and me and a teeny, tiny pension. Such good fortune. Once more, I felt blessed.

After I retired, Alex and I celebrated our 50th anniversary with a vow renewal. Family came from California, Texas, Florida, and Massachusetts. We danced and laughed and remembered that 50 years had passed since I saw the handsomest guy I'd ever seen walk into the cafeteria.

Our children are grown now, and our grandchildren are busy making their way in the world.

So, here I am, the raggedy-assed kid who ran into a library for sanctuary and came out knowing that even Ugly Ducklings can find family, wicked witches can be foiled, and Leif the Lucky was right. No matter what—sail on.

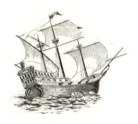

AFTERWORD

There is an apocryphal story, based on ancient lore, that the wounded warrior, in the course of healing, acquired a special wisdom about that process. I came to this business as many of us do, carrying wounds that needed healing. Early on, one of my mentors told me, "You can't send them [clients] where you haven't been." So, over the years, I made it a priority to immerse myself into my own healing.

Gestalt Therapy tapped into the disowned parts of me and fostered a level of integration that was a key stepping stone into wholeness.

Family Therapy gave me the tools and experience to begin to knit together broken bonds that had left me isolated and lonely. I learned to see how patterns of family behavior, which are almost as powerful as DNA, are passed through the generations. I found that, if I was very determined and lucky, I could try to change the course of my own family path. Once I understood this, I vowed that divorce and addiction would not be options for me. And so, I worked through the years, seeking treatment for my own addictive tendencies, immersing myself in trauma treatment and using every tool I could find so that the journey our children took could be vastly different than mine.

The teachings of Milton Erickson, founding president of the American Society for Clinical Hypnosis, had a deep influence on me. Although I didn't use classic hypnosis, I found his use of teaching tales and metaphor to be priceless tools to keep in my kit bag. And, thanks to the skill of my therapist, his stories helped me find my way back to myself.

When the Adult Children of Alcoholics movement began, I understood this was another path to healing the infection that spreads when one grows up in an alcoholic or addicted family.

The knowledge and skills base available now as therapeutic tools are way broader and varied than when I began my therapist's journey. For all whom I may have helped, I am so very grateful for your trust. For those whom I did not reach, I pray you found a way to win your freedom.

As you may have noticed in some of these stories, during times of great stress or crisis, I offered up the shortest prayer ever —*God, please help*—my heartfelt plea for divine intervention. God never failed to answer that prayer. Although I don't subscribe to a formal religion, I'm a true believer in a higher power who is always present and know that, in time, all my prayers will be answered.

CONTACT THE AUTHOR

I sincerely thank you for reading this book and hope you enjoyed it. I would be extremely grateful if you could leave a review on Amazon.

I'd love to hear your comments and am happy to answer any questions you may have. Do please get in touch with me by:

EMAIL: PINNYBUGAEFF01@GMAIL.COM

FACEBOOK: FACEBOOK.COM/PINNYBRAKELEYBUGAEFF

If you enjoy memoirs, I recommend you pop over to Facebook group We Love Memoirs to chat with me and other authors there.

FACEBOOK.COM/GROUPS/WELOVEMEMOIRS

I look forward to hearing from you.

Pinny Bugaeff

ACKNOWLEDGMENTS

I've been blessed with a number of people who have shown me love, kindness, and compassion, all of which helped fuel the writing of this memoir. Many of those early "angels" are long gone, but their gifts remain.

I thank my dad, who sang to me and taught me how to tell jokes; my mother, who endowed me with a huge helping of creativity; my great-grandmother, Gan, and Aunt Theresa, who spent hours reading me "just one more story"; Auntie May, my other mother, who always arrived just in time to take me back for a long visit in California where no one ever yelled; Miss Hallow, the library lady who made a story circle just for me; and Jeanie and Linda, friends who made me laugh and held me when I cried.

I thank my husband, Alex—best friend and listener; brainstorming, dishwashing, hand-holding lover—for walking through 54 years with me and for his continued encouragement to not only write, but to actually publish, this book.

I thank our son, Gregor, who continues to inspire me with his courage in daring to follow his muse, no matter where it takes him.

I thank our daughter, Mandy, and her husband, Mark, for

surrounding us with love and a generosity of spirit that sometimes brings me to tears.

And I thank Polly; you know you are not only The. Best. Sister. Ever. You are my funniest friend, designer whiz, and partner in crime. Love you to the moon and back.

I am blessed five times over with grandchildren— Hannah, Atticus, Finn, Sydney, and Eva. Funny and sweet and wise, they call me Peach and treat me like a rock star. Their parents and stepparents, some who grew up in similar swamps to me, are all accomplished and talented people—especially my darling niece, Kim—and find myriad ways to make sure I know I'm always surrounded by their circle of love.

From the bottom of my heart, I thank the pioneer therapists who shared their knowledge and professional expertise with me. They held my hand and passed me tissues as I waded through the long-ago battlefields of my past.

I thank the clients who sought me out and allowed me to join them on their journey. Your trust and courage have always been a source of inspiration. For those who did not find what you sought, I pray you found your way out of the shadows into the sunlight. I thank dear colleagues who marched with me through the trenches of human despair and taught me how to keep the faith.

Thanks to Dave and Billie Kapp, dear friends and travel companions, who gave me continued support to pursue my writing.

And last, but not least, thanks to my Friday morning toast group—Lisa, Jim, Paulette, Jackie, and Petie—friends for life.

Special appreciation to Victoria Twead and Jacky Donovan. When Ant Press gave me the opportunity to publish this book, you gave me a gift beyond pearls. Your expertise and loving kindness in editing and production was incredible. I think I'm the luckiest woman I know to have become a part of the "ant colony" you've created with Ant Press.

And, once more, I thank God for all He has given me, all He has taken away, and all that I am left with. I am truly blessed.

Made in the USA
Las Vegas, NV
09 August 2022